The sociology of health promotion

Over the last decade the promotion of health has become a central feature of health policy at local, national and international levels, forming part of global health initiatives such as those endorsed by the World Health Organisation. At the same time a concern with 'healthy living' has become a preoccupation for many people. *The Sociology of Health Promotion* responds by offering the first critical sociological account of these developments and locates them within a set of wider socio-cultural changes associated with late modernism. Drawing upon the work of Foucault, Beck, Giddens, Featherstone and others the book presents a theoretical as well as empirical examination of health promotion.

The Sociology of Health Promotion offers analyses of contemporary public health policy, lifestyle, consumption, risk and health. It also examines socio-political critiques of health promotion and reflects upon their implications for policy and practice. Substantive topics covered include: the institutional emergence of health promotion at both global and national levels, accidents and the risk society, smoking, HIV/AIDS, ageing, the body, and health-related consumption. A key theme of the collection is that health promotion is emblematic of wider socio-cultural changes. Changes such as the demise of institutional forms of welfare and social control, a blurring of 'expert' and lay knowledge, a heightened collective perception of uncontainable risks, and a shift to a consumer- rather than producer-driven economy.

This collection will be invaluable reading for students and social scientists with an interest in health and health policy, health promotors, public health doctors and practitioners engaging in critical reflection upon their professional activities.

Robin Bunton is Senior Lecturer in Social Policy at the University of Teesside, **Sarah Nettleton** is Lecturer in Social Policy at the University of York, and **Roger Burrows** is Reader in Sociology at the University of Teesside.

The sociology of health promotion

Critical analyses of consumption, lifestyle and risk

Edited by Robin Bunton, Sarah Nettleton and Roger Burrows

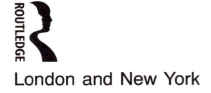

London and New York

First published 1995
by Routledge
11 New Fetter Lane, London EC4P 4EE

Simultaneously published in the USA and Canada
by Routledge
29 West 35th Street, New York, NY 10001

© 1995 Robin Bunton, Sarah Nettleton and Roger Burrows, selection and
editorial matter; individual chapters, the contributors

Phototypeset in Times by Intype, London
Printed and bound in Great Britain by
Biddles Ltd, Guildford and King's Lynn

British Library Cataloguing in Publication Data
A catalogue record for this book is available from the British Library

Library of Congress Cataloguing in Publication Data
A catalogue record for this book has been requested

ISBN 0–415–11646–5 (hbk)
ISBN 0–415–11647–3 (pbk)

Contents

Part III Knowledge, risk and health promotion

Part IV Health promotion, consumption and lifestyle

Illustrations

Contributors

Robin Bunton is Senior Lecturer in Social Policy in the School of Human Studies at the University of Teesside and is a member of the Centre for the Study of Adult Life (C-SAL) at the University.

Roger Burrows is Reader in Sociology in the School of Human Studies at the University of Teesside and is a member of the Centre for the Study of Adult Life (C-SAL) at the University.

Bruce Charlton works in the Department of Epidemiology and Public Health at the University of Newcastle upon Tyne.

George Davey Smith is Professor of Epidemiology at the University of Bristol.

Charlie Davison is a Research Fellow in the Department of Public Health at the University of Glasgow.

Norma Daykin works in the Faculty of Health and Community Studies at the University of the West of England, Bristol.

Jenny Douglas is Director of Health Promotion, Sandwell Health Promotion Unit.

Barry Glassner is a Professor of Sociology at the University of California at Los Angeles.

Judith Green is a Lecturer in Sociology at South Bank University in London.

Mike Hepworth is Reader in the Department of Sociology at the University of Aberdeen.

Peter Jackson is a postgraduate student in the School of Human Studies at the University of Teesside.

Michael P. Kelly is Professor of Social Sciences and Head of the School of Social Science at the University of Greenwich in London.

Jennie Naidoo works in the Faculty of Health and Community Studies at the University of the West of England, Bristol.

Sarah Nettleton is a Lecturer in the Department of Social Policy and Social Work at the University of York.

Martin O'Brien is a Lecturer in the Department of Sociology at the University of Surrey.

Richard Parish is Chief Executive of Humberside College of Health and Honorary Senior Fellow at the University of Hull.

Lindsay Prior is a Senior Lecturer in Sociology at the University of Ulster.

Nicki Thorogood is a Lecturer in Sociology at Guy's Dental School, United Medical and Dental Schools, in London.

Laurann Yen is Director, Primary Health Care, Tower Hamlets Healthcare Trust.

Acknowledgements

This volume presents chapters the bulk of which are substantially revised versions of papers that were first presented at a conference – *Towards a Sociology of Health Promotion and the New Public Health* – organised by the three editors at the University of Teesside under the auspices of the Centre for the Study of Adult Life (C-SAL) in September 1993. The book is the second to be derived from Teesside conferences concerned with the sociology of social and public policy and follows the earlier *Towards a Post-Fordist Welfare State?* (Routledge, 1994) edited by Roger Burrows and Brian Loader.

Thanks are due to all participants at the conference for making it such a stimulating affair, to Lesley Jones, and to colleagues from Teesside, especially Steven Muncer, Kate Gillen, Brian Loader and Mike Featherstone for their support, good humour and interest in our work over the last few years.

Special thanks should also go to Andrea Robinson, Elaine Hodgkinson and Ted Glover for their administrative support during a particularly difficult period in the early life of the School of Human Studies at Teesside.

This volume is dedicated to Jack Nettleton Burrows who was born in the month before it was completed.

Roger Burrows, Sarah Nettleton and Robin Bunton
York
October 1994

Chapter 1

Sociology and health promotion

Health, risk and consumption under late modernism

Roger Burrows, Sarah Nettleton and Robin Bunton

INTRODUCTION

During the last few decades inordinate attention has been paid to the promotion of 'healthy' living. This has come from governmental, academic, commercial and popular sources. Few people today can be unaware of the espoused merits of such a lifestyle. Anyone who has visited a supermarket recently, turned on the television, listened to the radio or read a magazine must have noticed that awareness of health issues is growing. Health is clearly a topical issue at both political and cultural levels.

At the political level from the mid-1970s, starting with *Prevention and Health: Everybody's Business* (DHSS, 1976a), there has been a dramatic increase in the number of policy documents and statements on prevention and, since the early 1980s, health promotion (see Parish, this volume, for a review). More recently a high profile has been given to *The Health of the Nation* (Department of Health, 1992a) and its attendant targets and to subsequent documents such as *Working Together for Better Health* (Department of Health, 1993a). It provides an interesting example of the 'globalisation' of policy and politics in that many of these documents and statements produced in Britain have drawn upon frameworks developed internationally by the World Health Organisation's *Health For All* (HFA) initiative. However, this said, such global initiatives may be interpreted very disparately by different nation states, and this process of policy mediation can tell us much about the policy and ideological priorities of different political regimes (Gustafsson and Nettleton, 1992).

At a cultural level 'healthism' has become a central plank of contemporary consumer culture as images of youthfulness, vitality, energy and so on have become key articulating principles of a range of contemporary popular discourses (Featherstone, 1991a; Savage *et al.*, 1992; Bunton and Burrows, this volume; Glassner, this volume; Hepworth, this volume). In the 1960s a list of 'health-related' commodities would have included items such as aspirins, TCP, Dettol and plasters. Today, however, it would include: food and drink; myriad health promoting pills; private health; alternative medicine; exercise machines and videos; health insurance; membership of sport and health clubs; walking boots; running shoes; cosmetic surgery; shampoo (for 'healthy looking hair'); sun oils; psycho-analysis; shell suits; and so on. The list is seemingly endless. Commodities have been 'transvalued' (Featherstone, 1991a) in two directions. First, some have been subject to a process whereby their original use value has been transformed into one increasingly articulated in terms of 'health' (for example, the 'greening' of household cleaning products, the shift from decorative to health-enhancing cosmetics and various forms of leisure). Second, and perhaps more significantly, some have been 'trans-valued' in the opposite direction, in that their original health use value has been transformed to take on a much wider social and cultural meaning (for example, running shoes, shell suits and body building).

Sociological analyses of health policy in general have, until recently, been a relatively neglected area of the sociology of health and illness (Gabe *et al.*, 1991; Stacey, 1991). Not surprisingly, then, this has also been the case in relation to health promotion (Thorogood, 1992b) and public health (Lewis, 1986) more generally. This book attempts to fill a gap in the literature by attempting to develop sociological perspectives and critiques of these key contemporary areas of health policy and practice.

HEALTH PROMOTION AND SOCIOLOGY

What is distinctive about health promotion is the attention that it gives to the *facilitation* of healthy lives: the idea that it is no good just telling people that they should change their lifestyles without also altering their social, economic and ecological environments. People must be *able* to live healthy lives. Health promotion aims to work not only at the level of individuals but also at the level of socio-economic structures and to encourage the creation and implementation of 'healthy public policies' such as those concerned with transport, environment, agriculture and so on.

We can see therefore that the promulgation of healthy lifestyles and the discourse of health promotion and the 'new public health' more generally are important and topical subjects which, although retaining some continuities with past health policy, can increasingly be viewed as representing a new paradigm of health care (Nettleton, 1995). Our con-cern in this volume is to try and make some sociological sense of health promotion and to review the critiques that are emerging in response to it.

So far sociologists have tended to contribute to the development and refinement of health promotion activities rather than analysing it as an object of inquiry. They have carried out surveys, interviews and obser-vations of people's lifestyles to provide information for health promotion campaigns. They have presented analyses of the aetiology and distribution of health and illness which reveal that adequate health policies must take structural and environmental factors into account. They have debated the political and ideological bases of health education and health promotion activities. Hitherto, however, what sociologists have failed to do is to adequately develop analyses of the phenomenon itself. Herein lies the rationale for this collection: how are we to account for and make sense of the rise of, and preoccupation with, the growing field of health promotion and, relatedly, the new public health?

The volume is largely the outcome of a conference held in September 1993 at the University of Teesside, organised by the editors, which aimed to address this question. Although the contributors were working on a disparate array of substantive areas within the field of health promotion many drew upon a common theoretical literature and a related set of conceptual concerns. This degree of theoretical and conceptual accord, which is also apparent in the chapters throughout this book, was not something that the conference organisers/volume editors had anticipated. Although the familiar sociological concerns with the social divisions of gender, sexuality, race, age and class are evident, it appears that sociologists also view health promotion as emblematic of wider contemporary social and cultural changes – changes which are characteristic of the acceleration of the processes associated with late modernity (Giddens, 1990; 1991), the rise of the risk society (Beck, 1992a; 1992b) and the growing preoccupation with the body, lifestyle and consumer culture (Featherstone, 1987; 1991a; 1991b; Featherstone *et al.*, 1991). As things currently stand the sociology of health promotion is a sociology of risk, knowledge, consumption, lifestyle, culture and, of course, health.

The dominant strand of the sociology of health promotion is its concern to analyse the phenomena as a characteristic of the much wider set of socio-economic and cultural processes associated with late modernism. As we approach the end of the millennium many sociologists have turned their attention to the dominant social formations that appear to be emerging. Many have conceptualised the changes taking place as being part of a process of *post*modernisation in which the social structures of modernity are superseded by radically new sets of arrangements (Lash and Urry, 1994). However, other writers, most notably Giddens (1990; 1991), argue that it is more appropriate to think about the contemporary period as being one in which, rather than being superseded, the central aspects of modernity are becoming significantly more dynamic and accentuated:

> The modern world is a 'runaway world': not only is the *pace* of social change much faster than in any prior system, so also is its *scope* and the *profoundness* with which it affects pre-existing social practices and behaviour.
>
> (Giddens, 1991: 16; emphasis in the original)

Giddens argues that it is therefore more appropriate to talk about the contemporary period as being one of *late* modernism. This implies that existing social relations and social structures are in an inherent state of flux. Social organisations are becoming increasingly subject to constant reorganisation and change and social life is becoming increasingly more reflexive. For example, it is claimed that we are witnessing the demise of traditional institutional forms of welfare and social control, a blurring of 'expert' and lay knowledge, a heightened collective perception of uncontainable risks, and a shift to a consumer- rather than producer-driven economy. This volume examines the manner in which some of these changes are manifesting themselves in health promotion and the new public health – central features of contemporary health policy.

The volume thus attempts to: develop contemporary sociological analyses of health promotion; develop analyses on matters in relation to health promotion which are of interest to contemporary sociology, including risk, the body, consumption, and processes of surveillance and normalisation; and develop critiques of health promotion which are of interest to health and medical practitioners, including issues of gender and race in the implementation of health programmes, cultural dimensions of lifestyles and health behaviours, and the marketing and consumption of health-related activities.

THE ORGANISATION OF THE VOLUME

The book is organised into four sections. The first provides an introduction to the institutional and policy context of health promotion activity in order to provide a backdrop against which the sociological analysis of the phenomena can be situated. The second assesses a range of socio-political critiques which have been made of health promotion from sociological, feminist, political and cultural perspectives. The third examines different aspects of health promotion in relation to the intersection of the sociology of risk and the sociology of knowledge. The fourth and final section examines health promotion in relation to the sociology of consumption and lifestyle.

The institutional context of health promotion

The institutional context of health promotion is examined at an international, national and local level. The chapter by Richard Parish traces the development of the rhetoric of health promotion by examining various policy documents and World Health Organisation (WHO) literature. The chapter provides useful details of the political and policy background of health promotion and suggests the likely future trajectory of its development. The chapter by Laurann Yen is, again, written from the perspective of the institutional context of health promotion, but this time at the more local level. She examines the development of health promotion in the light of the implementation of the internal market as part of the NHS reforms. She argues that initially there were indications of health promotion becoming more consumer oriented and market responsive under these new management arrangements. Latterly, however, there have been indications of a marked medical dominance and the introduction of provider-led surveillance oriented approaches. The chapter questions whether, despite the rhetoric, there has really been a significant change in perspective. Having set the institutional and policy context of health promotion the next section of the volume examines the various critiques that have been made of it.

Socio-political critiques of health promotion

Over the years social science in general, and medical sociology in particular, has provided many important critiques of various forms of health and medical care. In many respects health promotion has drawn upon these critiques as it has established itself as a practice distinct from systems of health care based upon the bio-medical paradigm. However, health promotion itself has not been immune from these critiques. In particular sociologists have pointed to the individualising tendencies in health education and promotion. The perpetuation of structural inequality by the use of value laden – sexist and racist – health promotion programmes has also been identified. Although structuralist critiques have formed the main critical platform in the sociology of health promotion more recently attention has been drawn to surveillance and consumption critiques – critiques developed throughout the present volume.

The chapter by Sarah Nettleton and Robin Bunton provides an overview of these existing sociological critiques of health promotion – structural, surveillance and consumption based. The chapter also identifies a number of substantive areas that have been explored by these analyses: populations, identities, risks and environments. In doing this it attempts to map out the existing terrain of the sociology of health promotion.

The chapter by Norma Daykin and Jennie Naidoo presents an overview of feminist critiques of health promotion. Different types of health promotion and a range of feminist perspectives are reviewed and then discussed in relation to each other. The chapter identifies how various feminist critiques offer insights at different levels of service provision. It argues that feminist perspectives are more developed in relation to the more authoritarian strategies which form the central planks of Government health promotion strategy. Feminist critiques of other, more collective forms of health promotion are also discussed. The chapter concludes that health promotion tends to take gender inequalities for granted and, in adapting strategies to the *status quo*, may be accused of actively reproducing these inequalities.

Many health promotion and public health strategies have been found to be not only sexist but also to be based on fundamentally racist assumptions. However, this has been a relatively neglected area in the academic literature on health promotion. Furthermore, at the level of practice the issue of race is also either neglected or presumed to be a matter of cultural difference rather than a matter of institutional and structural racism. Existing critiques in this field are reviewed and developed more fully in the chapter by Jenny Douglas.

The chapter by Michael Kelly and Bruce Charlton offers a polemic against many of the main strands of contemporary health promotion theory and practice. By drawing upon international, national and local level examples they argue that a range of tensions in the application of health promotion philosophy has become apparent. They argue that on the one hand, much health promotion is driven by a subjective and holistic notion of health, an emphasis on positive health, and a rejection of the biomedical model, but on the other hand, the epistemology and the WHO *Health for All* project remains vested in traditional expertise founded in technicist and scientific rationalities. These and other tensions are then theorised with reference to sociological debates concerning the modern, the postmodern and processes of postmodernisation.

The final chapter in this section, by Charlie Davison and George Davey Smith, examines the political critiques of health promotion implicit within many of the previous chapters. They point out that many of the recent debates about, and criticisms of, health promotion and the new public health appear to transcend conventional political boundaries between left and right. In some respects this leaves those working within the field with a sense of unease, in that they have lost any political direction or commitment. This political conundrum forms the focus of this chapter and suggestions about how we might not have to 'throw the baby out with the bath water' are outlined.

Knowledge, risk and health promotion

The third section of the volume examines various aspects of the relationship between knowledge (both 'lay' and medical), risk and health. The first chapter in this section, by Peter Jackson, examines the scientific basis of health promotion discourse by way of a case study of the social construction of the health effects of passive smoking within scientific research. By drawing upon the work of Ludwick Fleck, Jackson explores the emergence and development of the construction of passive smoking as a threat to public health. He challenges the assumptions of scientific realism and locates the production and content of this new medical knowledge in discourse and process.

The next two chapters in the section examine contemporary sociological perspectives on accidents. Accidents are the major cause of death for children and a significant cause of death, disability and distress for all age groups. Since the middle of the twentieth century there have been various initiatives aimed at reducing the death rate from accidental injury, culminating in Britain in 1992 with *The Health of the Nation* targets. In her chapter Judith Green argues that the accident prevention literature upon which such policies are based appeals to a discourse of risk assessment, which creates a world in which the risks of particular actions are known or knowable and in which all events are therefore preventable; accidents result not from random misfortune but from the miscalculation of risk. This risk assessment discourse creates the 'lay person' who emerges as the foil of the accident prevention professional and who persists in anachronistic beliefs in fate and luck when explaining accidents. The chapter examines some paradoxes at the heart of this discourse using data from a study on how accidents are constructed. It suggests that a focus on accidents as a category of misfortune, rather than an eclectic group of injuries, may explain the failure of accident prevention strategies.

Lindsay Prior, in his chapter, complements this argument. He begins with the observation in *The Health of the Nation... And You* (Department of Health, 1992b) that 'in theory at least, all accidents are preventable'. He argues that this notion of an accident as something calculable, controllable and therefore preventable carries within it some of the most fundamental themes of modernity. The chapter examines the modernist vision of chance, determinism and accidents and draws out the implications of that vision for health promotion programmes. In particular it focuses on the contradiction that exists between the understanding of accidents as things which happen to individuals, and the mathematical concept of an accident as a chance event in a population of events. It concludes with an examination of the causal logic that lies behind a number of official publications on accidents and accidental deaths.

The final chapter in the section, by Nicki Thorogood, is again concerned with the dynamics of modernity. However, this chapter examines the place of anti-rational discourses through an examination of the construction of safe dental practice. It is argued that such practice is constructed through the ways in which patients talk about 'risk' and 'fate' and by media reporting. The data examined come from a survey of public opinion on HIV and dental practice. Initial responses suggested a 'liberal' rational attitude which involves the calculation of risk and corresponding decision making. But a further examination of people's comments suggests that 'anti-rational' discourses such as 'trust' and 'morality' are central to the construction of safety in dental practice. The chapter concludes that popular discourse around HIV and dentistry highlights the fragility of rational discourse and the coexistence of contemporary anti-rational alternatives.

Health promotion, consumption and lifestyle

The fourth and final section of the volume examines various aspects of the relationship between health, consumption and lifestyle. The first chapter in this section is an extract from a book, *Bodies: The Tyranny of Perfection*, by the American sociologist Barry Glassner. The extract provides a number of interesting insights into contemporary American consumer culture in relation to the body and health. It provides an analysis of tendencies already becoming increasingly apparent within the context of Britain such as the growing popularity of cosmetic surgery and the growth of the 'diet industry'.

The chapter by Mike Hepworth further examines this theme by analysing the ageing body in the context of both the discourses of consumer culture and health promotion. Drawing on social problems theory, the chapter adopts a critical approach to the concept of 'positive ageing', defined in the gerontological literature as the promotion of a 'positive' attitude towards ageing and old age. Hepworth argues that 'normal' and 'abnormal' ageing are not objectively distinctive biological conditions waiting to be discovered once the appropriate empirical methodology has been refined, but are socially constructed moral categories which reflect the prevailing context of consumerism, decentralisation and voluntarism.

The chapter by Martin O'Brien examines the role that the concept of 'lifestyle' has played in the discourse of health promotion and the new public health. He argues that health promotion represents a critical moment of socio-political change in the organisation and control of health resources. He explores the politicisation of health through the fragmenting vehicle of lifestyle research programmes, behaviour regimes and health promotion schemes.

The final chapter, by Robin Bunton and Roger Burrows, attempts to explore the themes of health and consumption in the context of the interaction between the discourses of consumer culture and health promotion. It examines the relationship between health promotion and 'health-related' consumer culture in the context of case studies of both contemporary drug culture and middle class consumption patterns. It argues that in order to understand the emergence of health promotion it is necessary to situate it within contemporary consumption practices and that important aspects of its work only make sense in relation to late modern consumer culture.

CONCLUSION

The volume does not pretend to offer a definitive statement on the sociology of health promotion. It attempts, however, to illustrate that a sociology of health promotion is becoming an important project for contemporary sociology more generally. It seeks to clarify some of the main parameters of the field, critically review the existing literature in the area, and provides some examples of where a sociological analysis of health promotion might be developed. Finally, it provides a corrective to some of the more Utopian claims made by health promotion advocates and contributes to debates within health promotion itself. The concepts of health, risk and consumption are central themes of both contemporary sociology and health promotion. Our hope is that the volume will generate constructive debate both within and between the disciplines of health promotion and sociology around these and other concerns.

Part 1

The institutional context of health promotion

Chapter 2

Health promotion
Rhetoric and reality

Richard Parish

INTRODUCTION

Health and disease change with the times. At the turn of the century, ill-health patterns were determined largely by infectious diseases. Today, in western industrialised countries, they are distinguished mainly by the high incidence of chronic degenerative diseases, such as cardiovascular diseases and cancers. The social patterns of health related behaviours also change over time. In the United Kingdom, the rise and fall in smoking prevalence over the last hundred years, and a change in the nation's diet, are classic examples. In the last two decades, there has been an increasing recognition by policy makers that lifestyle and health are inextricably linked, and that in order to bring about improved prospects for health it is necessary to ameliorate the damaging effects of unhealthy lifestyles.

It was in this context that the World Health Organisation (WHO) launched its Health Promotion Programme in 1981. This established a set of concepts and principles which, WHO argued, should underpin all health promotion activities. The programme has received an overwhelming endorsement from the international community. This chapter provides a brief description of the emergence of health promotion at the level of both rhetoric and implementation.

THE EMERGENCE OF HEALTH PROMOTION

The term 'health promotion' was virtually unknown until the late 1970s. It reached remarkable prominence, however, in less than a decade, and now figures as a key policy issue on the agenda of many nations, particularly those in the Western, industrialised world. The United Kingdom has recently embraced the need for a new approach to health in a major White Paper, *The Health of the Nation* (Department of Health, 1992a). This builds upon the principles and approaches espoused by the WHO in its internationally endorsed *Health For All* programme (WHO Regional Office for Europe, 1985).

The notion of 'health promotion' had its origins in 1980 (Kickbusch, 1986). At that time, the WHO Regional Office for Europe was in the process of planning its health education programme for the period 1980 to 1984. There was a dawning recognition that health education in isolation from other measures would not necessarily result in the radical changes required to herald a new era of improved health. As a consequence, agreement was reached within the Regional Office to introduce a new programme that would address a range of non-educational approaches designed to improve the health prospects of the European Member States. This programme, designated 'health promotion', received the necessary political support to attract funding for its own designated staff and operational budget. It did not replace the existing health education programme, but acted in tandem with it.

In parallel with the WHO initiative, there was a growing recognition within the United Kingdom that traditional approaches to health education would not bring about the social changes necessary to secure a significant improvement in the population's health prospects. At a national level, the Health Education Council (1983) commissioned a confidential report on the additional measures necessary to complement its existing activities. At a more local level, a few individual Area Health Authorities were beginning to recognise that the translation of health knowledge into behavioural change required a more comprehensive approach than health education alone (see for example Stockport Area Health Authority (1980)).

In many ways the scene had already been set at a national level within the United Kingdom some four years earlier. In 1976 the Health Departments for England, Wales, Scotland and Northern Ireland published a major policy discussion document, *Prevention and Health: Everybody's Business* (DHSS, 1976a). Although this policy statement sought to achieve an important reorientation in the planning of health care in its broadest sense, it had not yet grasped the concepts and principles later to be embraced by the WHO. *Prevention and Health: Everybody's Business* shifted the health care debate away from treatment and towards prevention, but did not fully grasp the notion that health is created largely outwith the health care sector. Consequently, the document focused to a large extent on the provision of preventative services, such as screening, and the individual's responsibility to adopt healthy behaviour patterns. Indeed, the discussion paper explicitly ignored the influence of social and cultural factors with such statements as:

> many of the current major problems in prevention are related less to man's (*sic*) outside environment than to his own behaviour; what might be termed our lifestyle. For example, the determination of many to

smoke cigarettes in the face of the evidence that it is harmful to health and may well kill them.

(DHSS, 1976a:17)

The confusion of thinking in the mid- to late 1970s was exemplified extremely well in this DHSS document. Hard on the heels of such a dogmatic statement about personal responsibility, the paper continued with:

What is the role of Government in these matters? Is it largely the duty to educate, and to ensure that undue commercial pressures are not placed upon the individual and society? How far is the choice of the individual in these matters a free one and how can the individual be shown clearly the basis for the various options open to him so that he may make his choice with the greatest possible knowledge.

(DHSS, 1976:17)

And so the seeds were sown for what became a classic debate in the later 1970s and early 1980s: to what extent is the individual responsible for his or her own health, the so-called 'victim blaming' approach, and how far is health a collective responsibility to be addressed by communities and society as a whole.

Although *Prevention and Health: Everybody's Business* illustrated the flawed conceptual thinking of the time, it did stimulate a quality of debate that hitherto had been absent. Furthermore, it emphasised the inequalities in health that existed between different social groups, an issue which was to achieve great prominence within only a few years. First and foremost, it highlighted the geographical variation in mortality and demonstrated clearly that the South of England fared considerably better than the North East, Scotland and Wales. Perhaps even more noticeable than the geographical differences, the document commented on the marked variations between socio-economic groupings. Moreover, it observed that these had been apparent since the first data on social class were collected in the Census of 1911. It went on to highlight that the socio-economic variations in sickness were just as pronounced as those for mortality.

A plethora of Government policy documents and consultative papers during the late 1970s and early 1980s continued to set the climate for a more comprehensive approach to health promotion, albeit that national policy initiatives failed to demonstrate a genuine understanding of the underlying concepts and principles. They failed to recognise that the services provided by the health care system would have only a limited impact upon the health prospects of the population at large unless accompanied by a range of complementary socio-economic and environmental developments.

BEYOND THE UNITED KINGDOM

The United Kingdom was not alone in debating how best to improve health prospects in the last quarter of the century. Much of the industrialised world was considering how to address the ever increasing demands upon health care systems.

One of the most influential developments on the international scene during the 1970s was the publication of the Lalonde Report (Lalonde, 1974). Marc Lalonde was at that time the Minister for Health and Welfare in Canada. As the preface to his paper made clear, the time had come for a reassessment of Canada's approach to the future health and well-being of its citizens:

> Good health is the bedrock on which social progress is made. A nation of healthy people can do those things that make life worthwhile, and as the level of health increases so does the potential for happiness ... The health care system, however, is only one of the ways of maintaining and improving health ... For the environmental and behavioural threats to health, the organised health care system can do little more than serve as a catchment net for the victims ... The goal [of the Government of Canada] will continue to be not only to add years to life, but life to our years.

> (Lalonde, 1974:5)

The foundation stone of the Lalonde Report was an unequivocal questioning of the popularly held belief that the level of health equates to the quality and quantity of medical care. Although Lalonde highlighted the need for a more public health oriented approach to the future health of Canadians, ostensibly for altruistic reasons, a careful scrutiny of the proposals leads to the inevitable conclusion that economics was also a major consideration.

Lalonde stated that one of the major barriers to a more comprehensive analysis of the influences upon health was the absence of a conceptual framework. He argued that, without such a framework, it would be difficult to organise the various factors into manageable segments that would be amenable to analysis and evaluation. Lalonde insisted that policy makers required a 'map of the health territory'.

There is little doubt that the Lalonde report represents one of the milestones in the development of health promotion policy. Although born out of financial concerns, and operating on a medical model of prevention that today many would regard as outmoded, *A New Perspective on the Health of Canadians* was one of the first major governmental statements to recognise that maintaining the *status quo* in health care delivery was subject to the law of diminishing marginal returns. It can be criticised for paying too little attention to the impact of environment upon lifestyle without recognising, in effect, that lifestyle is the social aspect of the environment. Nevertheless, it was a bold political initiative which set new horizons for those involved in promoting the public's health. It had more impact outside Canada in terms of health policy development, however, than within it, partly due to the fact that it was a Federal Report and health is primarily a Provincial responsibility (Hancock, 1986). The mechanisms for implementation did not exist.

Canada, however, was not the only country reviewing its approach to public health at the end of the 1970s and during the 1980s. The United States and many other Western industrialised countries were following the same trail. In the Republic of Ireland, for example, the Minister of Health established a working group in 1985 with the specific remit to provide advice on the creation of a health promotion policy. As was the case with similar initiatives elsewhere, the Irish exercise was driven, at least in part, by economic considerations. The working group's recommendations, accepted by the Minister, were published in 1986 and defined health promotion as:

> The process which aims at improving the quality of life of the whole population no matter what a person's basic level of health. It is based on the understanding that health is more than an absence of disease and therefore is positive in concept.
>
> (Health Education Bureau, 1986:2)

The Irish report went on to comment that health promotion had its origins in the realisation that the major, modern day epidemics of cardiovascular diseases, cancers and accidents are associated with unhealthy behaviours and lifestyles. It did recognise that health promotion is broader than disease prevention and health education in that it accepted that those individuals who wished to adopt a healthier lifestyle may be constrained from so doing by environmental and socio-economic factors beyond their control. The report accepted that a coordinated strategy is required between Government, public sector departments and the public at large.

The aim of public policy initiatives to promote health, the report argued, should be: to add life to years by enabling as many people as possible to remain healthy and active throughout their lives; to add health to life by reducing the occurrence of illness and accidents; and to add years to life by increasing the average life expectancy of the individual.

The new conceptual thinking about health was also starting to have an impact during the mid-1980s in the Central and East European countries of the Soviet bloc. Hungary established a Committee in October 1986 chaired by the Deputy Prime Minister in response to the poor health status of the population by comparison with the European mean. Although recognising that the economic situation was not necessarily conducive to Government intervention in the cause of improved health, the Hungarian proposals clearly endorsed the view that the only logical response to the grave morbidity and mortality statistics would be a 'collective social responsibility' geared to action across the broad spectrum of sectors in the economy (Kokeny, 1987).

The strategy was debated and accepted at the 4 June 1987 session of the Council of Ministers, which endorsed the view that it was the Government's responsibility to create an economic climate that made health enhancing behaviour an easier choice for increasing numbers of people. The Hungarian proposals accepted that every state department had a role to play as they all helped to shape the societal context for health.

The strategy and plan of action agreed by the Hungarian Government were among the most comprehensive in Europe at that time. The programme is still to see the light of day, however, due to the preoccupation with an ailing economy suffering from the pangs of transition, the removal of key ministers and bureaucrats in the 1990 election, and the fact that the country's infrastructure is still in a state of flux.

RHETORIC RATHER THAN REALITY

Given the apparent political commitment to health promotion and a new vision of public health in so many countries, what lay behind the inability to translate policies into action? Like health promotion itself, the answer is almost certainly multidimensional.

First, change takes time. Establishing an agenda for innovation and development does not of itself ensure that implementation will automatically follow. The ideas will have to be acknowledged by the vast array of potential actors involved in health promotion and the consequences deduced. Indeed, those involved in planning programmes of health promotion recognise that it is essential to create a climate of opinion conducive to change well in advance of any attempt to implement the changes themselves (*Health Promotion International*, 1986; Parish, 1986). Moreover, governments are largely reactive to social movements rather than the stimulus for them. They need to feel secure in the knowledge that any significant shift in policy will be acceptable to the majority of the electorate. New ideas, therefore, frequently have a long gestation period to allow full consideration of the public's response. Providing that a full and comprehensive process for public consultation is actually in place, it could legitimately be argued that this is entirely consistent with the principle that advocates community involvement in the process of health promotion.

Progress is also hindered by changes in government administration, ministers and senior officials. By definition, the time-scale for health promotion, and the targets set for achievement, exceeds that of most governments. New administrations may not accept the commitments made by their predecessors, and even if they do, it takes time to come to terms with ministerial briefs and establish the political will to maintain progress.

It must also be acknowledged that the pressures on the health care system described earlier, in terms of both demand and finance, ensure that the curative services remain a priority. The Australian response to WHO's *Health For All* programme recognised that the orientation of the health system towards treatment and care results in the consequential neglect of prevention. Moreover, the Advisory Council to the Australian Health Ministers was honest enough to accept that bureaucracies and parliaments lack a sense of urgency when dealing with the prevention of chronic disease compared to their response to acute health problems (Australian Health Ministers' Advisory Council, 1988).

Finance is also clearly a barrier to change, although this may be more of a perception than a reality. The health care system is so preoccupied coping with the demand for its curative and rehabilitative services that it is difficult to bring about the reorientation that is embodied in the principles of health promotion. Within the United Kingdom for example it has been argued that short-term economic considerations have led to the comparative neglect of the long-term strategic objectives of the National Health Service (Ham, 1984). Furthermore, the 'pay off' in terms of reduced demand, is perceived as being long term, usually longer than the lifetime of the government of the day. This is despite the fact that the evidence indicates that much health promotion activity is cost effective (Godfrey *et al.*, 1989).

The complexity of coordination is a further barrier to policy implementation. Not only does health promotion require a commitment across most government departments and many sectors of the economy, it also requires action at every level: local, regional and national. Coupled with the potential for conflicts of interest, such as the perceived reduction in tax income and possible unemployment in the tobacco industry as a result of a lower cigarette consumption, the issue is clearly one of great complexity.

The above may give some indication of the constraints imposed at the point of translating policy into practice. Perhaps the greatest barrier of all, however, is that the actual strategies devolving from the laudable policy statements of countries around the world would indicate that a clear vision of health promotion in practice has been somewhat lacking.

HEALTH PROMOTION AND THE WORLD HEALTH ORGANISATION

It was against the background of escalating demands for health care caused by lifestyle related ill health, and the political imperative to reassess the notion of preventative medicine and health education, that health promotion as it is understood in the 1990s was born. Although the political context was provided by its member states, there is little doubt that the WHO took on the leadership role. It did so through two specific initiatives, namely the development of *Health for All by the Year 2000*, and the complementary Health Promotion Programme.

The Thirteenth World Health Assembly meeting in May 1977 acknowledged that despite the resources devoted to the health care system and technological developments since the end of the Second World War people's health status was lower than might have been expected. Moreover, massive inequalities in health still existed, not only between nation states, but also across different groups within countries. Consequently, the World Health Assembly adopted a major new programme, *Health for All*, in an effort to remedy these concerns. In so doing, the Assembly endorsed the view that this should be the main social target of both government and the World Health Organisation.

Further support for WHO's *Health for All* (HFA) programme was also forthcoming in the following year. On 12 September 1977, a major international conference held in Alma Ata in the Soviet Union issued a declaration on primary health care. This resulted in global support for the proposals, which adopted a broad definition of health and primary health care (WHO, 1978). The Alma Ata declaration endorsed the view that health is more than the absence of disease or infirmity; it is the attainment of the highest possible level of health as an important social goal. Not only is it a fundamental human right, but it requires a concerted effort by 'other social and economic sectors in addition to the health sector'.

In Europe, most countries had drawn up HFA proposals by the end of the decade. Whilst not establishing a specific HFA strategy, the United Kingdom agreed to monitor progress towards HFA targets. The Government argued that its health care policy overall was distilled in its statement in 1981, *Care in Action* (DHSS, 1981), and that there were specific initiatives in various disease prevention and health promotion areas, such as HIV and AIDS, non-smoking and accident prevention. In its second monitoring report to WHO, the UK Government stated that the major thrust of health policy remained unchanged since 1981, although there had been some sharpening of focus in areas such as health promotion, disease prevention and primary health care. With regard to equity, the report confirmed that resources were being reallocated to those parts of the country most disadvantaged in terms of standardised mortality ratios.

Although there was no formal HFA strategy, it was argued that the Government fully endorsed the principles and ensured that all the major components were reflected in policy formulation. The United Kingdom response pointed out that the maximum freedom is given to local Health Authorities, but the planning guidelines issued by the Department of

Health incorporated HFA strategic thinking. However, according to Turner (1986) in an article in the *Times Health Supplement*, only eight of the fourteen NHS Regions had set targets or earmarked funds for prevention and health promotion by 1986.

The fact that this resulted in criticism by the Public Accounts Committee may well have been one of the key pressures for further action. However, not until June 1991 did the UK publish a national health strategy for England (Department of Health, 1991). This was in the form of a comprehensive consultation document, and sought reaction and comment from a wide section of the British public and commercial life.

Wales, Scotland and Ireland have separate planning mechanisms for health, and it was Wales that produced the first population health strategy within the UK (Health Promotion Authority for Wales, 1990). Both the Welsh and English strategies stressed the need for multisectoral collaboration in order to tackle the fundamental influences upon lifestyle-related health and disease.

CONCEPTS AND PRINCIPLES

There seems little doubt that HFA provided the context for WHO's health promotion programme to become established and to flourish. In many ways, this programme has added substance to the more esoteric HFA proposals. Although it had its origins in 1980, from the point of view of funding, the health promotion programme began life in January 1984 as part of the seventh general programme of work of the WHO Regional Office for Europe. However, the preparatory work had commenced some four years earlier when a study was commissioned to determine the meaning of the term 'health promotion' in Europe, from both theoretical and practical standpoints.

In preparation for the concepts and principles document (WHO, 1984) WHO commissioned a technical paper which reviewed the current situation (Anderson, 1983). The following definition for health promotion attracted widespread support:

> Any combination of health education and related organisational, political and economic intervention designed to facilitate behavioural and environmental adaptations which will improve or protect health.
>
> (Anderson, 1983:11)

Five key principles were described in the final document (WHO, 1984).

1 Health promotion involves the population as a whole and the context of their everyday life, rather than focusing on people at risk for specific diseases.

2 Health promotion is directed towards action on the determinants or causes of health.
3 Health promotion combines diverse, but complementary, methods or approaches.
4 Health promotion aims particularly at effective and concrete public participation.
5 Health professionals, particularly in primary health care, have an important role in nurturing and enabling health promotion.

The range of methodologies described in the document includes not only education and mass communication (the health education component) but also legislation, fiscal measures in the form of either subsidies or taxation, organisational change, and community development. It requires the involvement, therefore, of most sectors of economic and social activity, hence the emphasis on health promotion being a government led exercise, both locally and nationally.

The WHO (1984) team also deliberated on the focus for health promotion; what should be the subject areas for attention? They concluded that there were five fundamental issues deserving of action:

1 Improving access to health.
2 The development of an environment conducive to health.
3 The strengthening of social networks and social supports.
4 Promoting positive health behaviour and appropriate coping strategies.
5 Increasing knowledge and disseminating information.

The access to health issue is concerned essentially with improving the opportunities to live a healthy lifestyle for everyone. It addresses the question of inequalities in health. Health promotion, therefore, should focus attention on the inequities which exist between different social groups to ensure that those currently disadvantaged have the same opportunities as the most advantaged.

The document further identified a number of potential dilemmas with which health promotion might have to contend. There is always the possibility of health promotion being viewed as 'healthism', with the public feeling that those responsible for health promotion are in the business of prescribing a particular way of life. Furthermore, health promotion programmes may be inappropriately directed at individuals, the so-called 'victim blaming' approach so apparent in many policy documents, rather than tackling the fundamental economic and social influences upon health. Moreover, resources, including education and information, may not be equally accessible to all people and in ways which are sensitive to their expectations and values, thereby exacerbating social inequalities. Furthermore, raising awareness without also increasing people's control of the determinants of health could be counterproductive. There is also the danger of professionalisation as the research base and theoretical frame-works for health promotion develop. Health promotion must not become an exclusive professional discipline, possibly operating to the exclusion of the public, although those who act on the public's behalf should be professional in their approach. 'Professionalism' rather than 'professional-isation' should be the goal.

CONCLUDING COMMENT

Most important of all of the developments over the past two decades has been the emergence of health promotion as a concept that has shifted the thinking of political decision makers away from individual and towards collective responsibility. In the words of Hafton Mahler in his last major speech as Director General of WHO:

> Health is indivisible ... the domain of personal health over which the individual has direct control is very small when compared to the influence of culture, economy and environment.

Chapter 3

From Alma Ata to Asda – and beyond

A commentary on the transition in health promotion services in primary care from commodity to control

Laurann Yen

INTRODUCTION

The title of this chapter reflects the emergence, through the introduction of the General Practitioner (GP) contract in 1990, of an approach to health promotion which encouraged United Kingdom health promotion services and activities to be seen as health commodities by the users, providers and purchasers of these services. Through these developments good health began to be approached as an 'elective' state, which could be achieved and enhanced by a range of consumer activities which directed the individual towards being more healthy. Such an approach encouraged users and providers to adopt a 'pick and mix' approach and is consistent with a rhetoric of consumer empowerment and involvement – principles of the 'new public health' that were laid out in the Alma Ata Declaration (WHO, 1978). It is also consistent with the philosophy of the NHS reforms which included the *New GP Contract*, in appearing to encourage a greater range of choices for individuals in their health care, and a greater level of individual responsibility for health status.

However, after less than two years of operation, changes were made to the regulations surrounding health promotion in primary care. A second GP health promotion contract was introduced in 1993 using a fundamentally different approach. The key elements of the new contract moved away from health and health promoting activity as commodities and began to reflect an increasingly pervasive managerialist approach for both professionals and consumers. It moved towards the identification and analysis of risk factors as the foundation for health promotion activity. This approach raises questions about the use of health promotion activity in primary care, the relationship between the consumer and the professional and between primary care and the new purchasers of health care – the District Health Authorities (DHAs).

THE 1990 HEALTH PROMOTION CONTRACT

The introduction of the *New GP Contract* in 1990 coincided with the transformation of Family Practitioner Committees into Family Health Services Authorities (FHSAs). The new FHSAs, themselves fledgling organisations, took on the task of introducing the principles of the NHS reforms into the primary care sector. This resulted in a move towards a more directly managed service. An indication of this type of change had been given in 1986 with the publication of *Primary Health Care: An Agenda for Discussion* (DHSS, 1986) which created the framework for bringing general practices in as a part of the 'managed' NHS as hospitals and community health services had been following the introduction of general management in 1984.

The 1990 contract for primary care included the introduction of two specific approaches to health promotion and illness prevention activity. First, as part of the new contract GPs were to receive additional remuneration for collecting and recording information on height, weight, blood pressure and urinalysis on each newly registered patient, and for inviting people on their list between 16 and 74 who had not consulted a doctor within the previous three years for a check-up. While this information was recorded by the practice, there was no requirement either to achieve a target coverage, to aggregate the information across the practice to develop a profile of its population, or to make any information gained more widely available to add to the knowledge of the local population. This last point created substantial tensions between primary care and the newly operational commissioning DHAs who, charged with assessing need across their resident populations, faced an information gap which they believed could be reduced by freedom of access to such information held by general practitioners. In retrospect, the introduction of such 'non-contributory' data collection enabled the principle of behavioural management to be reinforced without the immediate threat to professional autonomy, or the 'transformation of the caring function into an activity of expertise' (Castel, 1991: 290). Otherwise, this principle might have been seen as a direct challenge to the assumed confidentiality, integrity and inviolability of the doctor-patient relationship.

There were doubts expressed about the usefulness of patient data collection and three-year checks, from GPs and others. Those in the primary health care sector were left in no doubt over the Government's intention to give them more responsibility for preventing illness and promoting health. These changes, along with the direct link between performance and financial reward, laid the foundations for the further development of those principles in the 1993 health promotion contract.

The second element of health promotion activity in the 1990 contract was the introduction of funded health promotion clinics, which were new to primary care and which became a site for the development of health products. The clinics encouraged users, providers and purchasers to treat health as a highly manageable state which could be reached by the use of such products.

Health promotion clinics

The health promotion clinics were something of a surprise, and became an unusual area of innovation and expansion in the primary care sector. Under these arrangements general practices were enabled to apply for health promotion funds from the FHSA to support activities in primary care. The principal condition which governed approval was holding a clinic, or activity for ten people for a health promotion service agreed by the FHSA. This would then generate a fixed fee of £45 for the GP who ran the clinic, or under whose auspices the clinic would be run. The response which this produced was a proliferation of health promotion services for which approval was sought, and as a result new sets of health products were provided by a range of health care professionals which were made available to practice populations. The way in which these activities were introduced and used reinforced the idea of health as a commodity and was consistent with, and based on, the market principles and business ethos which had been brought into the health service through the NHS reforms.

One-stop services

The new health promotion clinics were a key element in the development of 'all under the one roof' services in general practice. This develop-ment was particularly welcomed by GPs themselves, many of whom were moving out of Health Authority owned health centre accommodation which they had shared with community health services into purpose-built practice premises. The availability of mechanisms like the cost rent scheme enabled this to occur without the GPs having to face high levels of financial risk. At the same time, the new NHS trusts began to seek to minimise their capital assets in order to reduce the capital charge of 6 per cent that was to be introduced. This changed the focus for the delivery of primary care and community health services in many areas from one dominated by the shared 'Community Health Centre' to one dominated by the general practice and its premises. GPs were keen to provide as many services as possible from the practice base and to extend services into new areas.

As part of their new contract, GPs were required to develop infor-mation leaflets and practice brochures which outlined the services they would provide to their patients. For the first time, patients were presented with a collection of information that would enable them to see what services were available to them, without the intermediation of the practice staff to provide an interpretation or a block to access. Many GPs were concerned about competition between practices for patients who might be influenced by the range of services provided on site and began to seek ways of increasing them, and making their practice more attractive. The reforms had introduced mechanisms to make it easier for patients to change their general practice, so GPs hoped both to attract new patients, and to keep existing patients, through the level and quality of, but also the ease of access to, services which patients might want or need to use. Health promotion clinics were a major part of these developments and encouraged both the practice and the patient to view health care options as items on a health care menu. To support this approach GPs and particularly GP fundholders sought to develop on-site services provided directly by practice staff, services which had been and often still were provided by community health staff in health centres, and new or additional services.

Cash and competition

One of the reasons for the expansion in range and number of health promotion activities in primary care was the fact that the funding to support the clinics was not cash limited – a fact not consistent with the increasingly dominant 'business culture' in the NHS. Nor was it consistent with the increasing emphasis on managerialism in primary care services. However, it played a highly significant role as a 'loss leader' in setting the framework for the future.

At the time, the lack of a cash limit encouraged an expansion of activity, providing additional income and hence greater buying power to the practices themselves and then to the other services/professionals from whom they themselves purchased health promotion services. The regulations enabled an unusual and compelling combination to occur: the NHS imperative – free at the point of delivery combined with the marketing of an unrationed range of new health products.

Because the clinics were not cash limited, the opportunity existed for services to develop without the usual need to compete for resources, or to argue for the need to increase them. The NHS Hospital and Community Health Services were beginning to see the impact of the NHS reforms with the introduction of the internal market. Service specifications created the basis for the development of the 'health product' – one which would be determined by the purchaser and which would be required to conform to a range of standards related to content, quality and price. Purchasers were either the DHA, who had most of the purchasing power, the newly introduced GP fundholders and, to a more limited extent, the

FHSAs. The new health promotion arrangements provided one of the main areas for the FHSA to act as a purchaser and to shape the nature of services offered in primary care. GPs, and particularly fundholding GPs, were keen to increase the range of services provided. Community Health Services and acute services providing services in primary care were keen to find new markets for their services to safeguard income levels threatened by the capacity of purchasers to contract with other providers, including those operating in the independent sector.

The introduction of the health promotion clinics, by providing a flexible, loosely controlled and open-ended resource, supported the interests of each of the key participants: for general practice in developing a one-stop comprehensive service; the FHSA in demonstrating its role as a serious manager and purchaser within the framework of the reforms; and for NHS providers in securing markets and income for their services/products.

Competition between each of the participants was to a large extent avoided because of the high degree of complementarity between their roles, and the lack of need to make prioritising decisions for funding. This was a period in which rising demand, accompanied by open-ended resources, led to an expansion both in the range of services/products provided and in the range of professionals involved in providing them.

Product development and marketing

Provided ten people could be gathered together in the name of health promotion, it was possible to apply for approval for a clinic. As the FHSAs were keen to promote both their own managing role in primary care and their purchasing role to develop primary care services, this led to a generally positive and imaginative approach being taken, where the FHSAs, as well as GPs and NHS providers, were able to foster new ideas for services in primary care.

GPs and other service providers had often felt frustrated by existing levels and types of service and by the difficulty encountered in attracting the resources to develop new services, particularly in primary care. The health promotion clinics gave the opportunity to address some of these issues and to extend the capacity of the primary care services. The choice of the clinics developed was not generally based on a comprehensively researched knowledge of the specific needs of the practice population, nor was their content, in general, rigorously assessed, as GPs and others sought to put in place the services which they had been unable previously to support. The resulting product mix reflected, as had often been the case with health education, the *interests and beliefs* of the clinical professionals about the needs of the population. The services which developed were not strongly linked to the existing health promotion or health education services, but were often used to broaden the clinical and educational services provided by the practice, and concentrated predominantly on identified diseases and disease processes. Health promotion clinics provided the umbrella for a range of 'secondary' care services, such as counselling, physiotherapy, chiropody and psychology, to enter the practice, which broadened the base from which these services were provided and increased their visibility within the primary care market.

The management of chronic illnesses such as diabetes and asthma began to be addressed more comprehensively with the introduction of the health promotion clinics as primary care services began to provide a more focused and comprehensive approach to continuing care. The development of protocols for care, which outlined the roles and responsibilities across all sectors, has been one result. Protocols, however, now act as product specifications for the management of these and other chronic illnesses, and reinforce the business culture introduced with the NHS reforms. New products also emerged which attempted to address the particular needs of local practice populations and sub-populations. Screening for diabetic retinopathy, travel clinics in areas where people frequently returned to their country of origin, menopause clinics, clinics which promoted exercise and the use of local sports and leisure facilities are examples of health care staff tailoring health promotion products to match the requirements of specific groups. The range of services of many practices extended well beyond those which had previously been provided, either separately or in partnership with community and other health services.

These services were marketed to the practice population in a number of ways. The increasing range of services offered by practice staff, and particularly the practice nurses, provided opportunities for direct recommendations or referrals to individual services. This applied principally to the secondary care services, such as physiotherapy, and to those services established to address specific diseases – heart disease, diabetes and asthma most frequently. People responding to the invitation for a three-yearly check, or newly registering with the practice might also be directed to health promotion options. Outside these areas, patients were encouraged through mostly practice-generated and practice-located information and services to 'get fit', 'stop smoking', 'lose weight', 'learn to relax' or 'eat right', all offering the opportunity to improve health and wellbeing through the consumption of these readily available healthy options.

Health promotion clinics were not aggressively marketed and frequently encountered the same problems as groups that were run by health promotion and health education services in other sectors, such as falling numbers and irregular attendance. Outside the main disease areas, little targeting of activity occurred, which increased the sense that these services were 'optional extras', or health accessories chosen by the patient either alone or on the advice of a health professional in the practice. Because the information was available mainly through the practice itself, or by word of mouth, there was little attempt to address the needs of patients who were not regular users of the practice.

Attempts were made to target or limit the use of the secondary services by negotiating criteria for access with the professional providers of the services. This did not, however, lead to more appropriate choices being made by the consumer, but to a new set of rules for entry to the system. Some tensions began to occur when the demands of the purchaser – usually the GP – for the service provided differed from the service which the provider thought appropriate. The pressure on these services was on the availability of appropriately tailored staff; while GPs and FHSAs had resources to enable them to purchase, the NHS services were not always able to provide the additional services without creating shortages of skill and time in other areas. This led quite quickly to the use of independent sector services, generally on a sessional basis, and reinforced the market-driven approach. Therapy services were the most common, with chiropody, physiotherapy and counselling services leading the way. These services similarly were not marketed aggressively to the practice population, but began to be seen as part of the 'menu' or 'repertoire' of services which a good practice could make available to its patients. The real or perceived benefits of access to these services was not widely explored, and multidisciplinary clinical audit of these primary care services had not yet been introduced.

There were, however, objections to the commodity approach to health promotion, most often from clinical professionals who feared both that those elements of their work that they considered to be most important would be lost to the time demands of less important work and that their clinical and professional autonomy would be threatened by the increasingly specific demands of patients and purchasers. Good examples of this can be seen in chiropody services. Some practices and FHSAs negotiated chiropody time as part of health promotion clinics, which made chiropody services widely available to all patients, not just those in 'priority' groups such as the elderly and diabetics. The service was marketed to patients through practice information, and then quickly through word of mouth. Because the service was marketed as available, the chiropodist had little power to exercise clinical judgement and to prioritise the workload – the service quite quickly became saturated.

At the end of the first year of the health promotion clinics a number of features of the new system could be discerned: health promotion clinics had become an integral part of the practice services; FHSAs were approving and resourcing a wide range of primary and secondary prevention and health promotion activities which had not previously been practice based; professionals were moving into primary care with an extended product range of services, from both the NHS and the independent sector; competition on the basis of price began to occur – examples of particular note were psychology and counselling services as well as NHS and private sector chiropody and physiotherapy; GPs, particularly in larger and fund-holding practices, were using extended ranges of practice-based services to improve practice image and competitiveness; practice patients were encouraged to take advantage of practice-based health promotion services in a 'pick and mix' way; secondary services, such as physiotherapy, were marketed as locally available (and quickly), generating patient approval and satisfaction; practice patients were encouraged to view clinics/activities as commodities which would enable them to feel more healthy; and costs kept on rising.

By 1992 it was clear that the open-ended approach which characterised the introduction of health promotion clinics was not going to continue. Three main concerns emerged. First, the cost of expanding and resourcing clinics continued to rise. Far from general practices introducing and monitoring services which they would personally provide, a proportion of health promotion monies was going to fund the services of a wide range of health care and health-related professionals. These providers in turn were encouraged by the initial success of their new ventures to continue to explore alternatives to traditional means of service provision and this increased the demand for further resources via approvals of new clinics. The lack of control over expenditure had introduced the notion of potentially unlimited product choice, and raised the expectations of both service providers and service users for freely available health commodities. These products differed from free access to the hospital-based disease orientated services which fall into the category of services for which, currently, the NHS is seen to have a responsibility. The new products were not primarily focused on treatment and cure, and were much more under the control of the user. The NHS was not used to funding such services nor to calculating the trade-off between the long-term health and social costs of an unhealthy community in comparison with the short-term costs of funding health promotion.

Second, with health promotion clinics offering a free choice of options to the service users, and operating as patient-generated choices, concern arose over the content and scope of the activities provided through NHS funding. If the service specification is largely determined by the individual user and provider, will the activities demanded be consistent with those thought appropriate for the NHS to provide? Will the NHS be funding activities or services which ought, properly, to be purchased by individuals? When does a health promoting activity move from the realm of individual choice to one in which the state recognises a responsibility? If the NHS itself actively markets a view about healthy lifestyles and behaviours and seeks to encourage individuals to adopt this view, where does responsibility for enabling this fall? The diversity of the activities and services provided through the health promotion clinics was repeatedly challenged as addressing the particular demands of individuals (as in the case of travel clinics), or niche markets (such as menopause clinics), or as of unproven, often of dubious, value.

Third, the lack of emphasis on outcome, either in clinical or economic terms began to be of concern. GPs were required to ensure that evaluations of clinics were conducted, but the nature and content of these evaluations were generally very loosely controlled. As a result, evaluations tended to reflect the mechanics of the process rather than the outcome of the activity. There was no attempt or requirement to assess the value, in economic terms, of the activities provided, nor any comparative assessment between services offered.

This is not to suggest that evaluation of outcome or value for money in clinical/health gain terms was widely used in the hospital sectors, nor that hospital sector services were demonstrably more effective. Indeed, health promotion clinics would be exceptional within the NHS if they were able to demonstrate a high degree of both clinical and economic effectiveness. The crucial differences that existed between the two sectors was the lack of a cash limit for the health promotion clinics, and the relatively higher degree of consumer involvement and choice they allowed. The culture of the managed market introduced into the NHS existed uneasily alongside the highly deregulated, open choice commodities approach represented by the free market in health promotion clinics.

MAKING THE TRANSITION

The new health promotion contract introduced in 1993 offered a profoundly different approach to the 1990 contract by: changing the perception of health promotion activity in primary care from healthy products to programmes; increasing the emphasis on managerialism in the primary care sector; and introducing a population risk and risk management approach into the primary care health promotion contract.

From products to programmes

The new contract introduced a practice programme of health promotion for which individual GPs would receive remuneration at a fixed rate. Rather than using the £45 per clinic model of the first contract, GPs were paid individually for an agreed programme of work. Programmes were to be based on three levels of activity or 'bands', with the most lucrative requiring a combination of data collection, risk identification and targeted intervention relating to coronary heart disease and/or stroke. The whole range of health promotion products which had been developed and made available was no longer to be funded. Transitional arrangements would enable a small number of activities to continue when they could be demonstrated to be 'worthwhile' but on the whole, the web of practice-based health promotion activity operating in primary care was likely to be dismantled. The change in the funding process was fundamental to the change in approach. All of those services that had been locally marketed as health-giving products – the counselling services, back care clinics, healthy eating, relaxation and well person services as well as those directly related to existing disease such as diabetes and asthma, like footcare and screening for diabetic retinopathy – would no longer be independently and individually funded.

Williams *et al.* (1993) suggest that the increase in the fee for the service element in GP reimbursement, which was the mechanism for funding the 1990 arrangements, might lead to an increased range of preventive services being made available, but a reduction in the quality of the primary care consultation. The implementation of the 1990 contract may have avoided some of the loss of quality issues by making extensive use of other professionals to provide the services. The degree to which these services could be defined as primarily preventive is open to debate, but perhaps to no greater extent than would have been the case if GPs themselves had undertaken the activities.

The introduction of the 1993 contract is far more likely both to reduce the range of services offered, and, by paying the GPs personally and directly, reduce the breadth of activity and specialist skills available to the practice population from professionals whom the practice no longer feels able to afford. In addition, the specific concern raised by Williams and his colleagues, that general GP consultations would be of lower quality because of the time devoted to income-generating health promotion is now perhaps of greater significance. In fact, substantial elements of the health promotion programme are carried out by practice nurses, who are also attempting to take up provision of some of the services previously offered. Fundholding practices may have more scope to continue to offer the range of services because of the flexibility available in the fund. The result for both fundholding and non-fundholding practices will be an approach to health promotion that will be more limited in content and professional input and in which the users will have fewer options from which to choose and fewer areas of health gain to explore.

More management

The 1993 contract introduced a highly structured accountability process for health promotion programme 'bandings'. The objectives of the new scheme were stated as being: to give a framework of national and local priorities for GP health promotion in England, informed by the *Health of the Nation* White Paper; greater flexibility for practices to develop their new approaches; better targeting of resources; wider access to health promotion for all patients; and better year-on-year control over expenditure (General Medical Services Committee, 1993).

A distinction was drawn between programmes for two chronic conditions, diabetes and asthma, and health promotion activity directed towards coronary heart disease (CHD) and stroke, which were the only two areas of health promotion activity which would continue to attract funding, and then on the basis of the programme submitted by the practice.

Practitioners would be required to demonstrate compliance with the guidance in order to obtain approval by satisfying that their proposed programme: met the content requirement for each banding and/or met the specific content requirement for chronic disease programmes; met the criteria that the programme was in accordance with modern medical opinion; and met, in the case of health programmes, an acceptable population coverage level.

Each requirement was accompanied by a strengthening of the managerial influence on primary care, and the increasing accountability of the GP, by setting out a complex and detailed approval and monitoring framework. Intense discussions were held to interpret some of the requirements. How would the financial allocation be derived if different partners in a practice applied for approval for different programmes? How was a non-smoker to be defined? Why was the recording process out of step with the national *Health of the Nation* data collection format? Each of these questions reflected some of the anxieties that had been generated by the less rigorous monitoring demands of the first contract, but also the impact of a much more structured accountability framework on the workload of a general practice whose available resources might well reduce. The stricter accounting and monitoring requirements has created pressure on practice data collection systems, and particularly on the practice nursing staff without necessarily addressing the benefits to be achieved. The content of the programmes provided was also prescribed through guidance contained in *Better Living – Better Lives* (NHS Management Excecutive, 1993) and specific guidelines relating to the management of asthma and diabetes, which restricted rather than enhanced the practices' capacity to develop their own approach despite the guidance stating the need for a more flexible approach.

Finally the 1993 contract introduced new performance measures for health promotion, which required the practice not only to collect data on those patients who came to the surgery, but to extend this coverage to reach practice registrants who were not regular attenders. This represents a shift in the nature of the relationship between the doctor and the patient from one of patient initiated (and therefore to at least some extent patient controlled) to one in which the GP actively seeks contact to fulfil a performance requirement.

The performance expectation rises to a maximum of 90 per cent coverage for the measurement and recording of blood pressure, whilst 80 per cent coverage of smoking status is expected and 75 per cent for body mass index, alcohol use and family history. This creates a contract which uses highly defined performance parameters on a narrow field of activity, with an increasing management of the process. The increasing rigour has not deterred GPs from applying for the maximum programme responsibility. For example, in a number of regions 90 per cent and above of practices obtained approval for a Band 3 programme (the highest paid) along with chronic disease management clinics. This may relate to the trade-off between loss of earnings and greater accountability where practices will accept a much higher level of external managerial control in order to maintain this level of income, but then use internal management measures, such as reliance on employed staff, to reduce the impact on the GP.

Risk

Alongside the increased managerial intervention in the process of providing health promotion services, the content of the 1993 contract was centred on the identification and targeting of 'risk' within the practice population. The risk factors especially targeted relate to CHD and strokes. The data collected ranged from smoking incidence in the practice population to information on blood pressure, weight, alcohol use and personal and family history of CHD and stroke. Interestingly, and inexplicably, the definitions used to report incidence are flexible, with practices asked, for example in the case of raised blood pressure, to indicate whether they use a different definition from that of the World Health Organisation (WHO).

At the same time as practices were being set performance measures for coverage, the individual user is being assessed on his or her performance as a 'healthy' individual – but only in relation to CHD and stroke. While there is no dispute about the importance of these conditions as major causes of death and debilitation, the concentration on risk factors associated with them creates a framework for the regulation of and intervention in an individual's health principally in relation to those conditions. It also implies an understanding of the individual based around the collection of particular risk factors they display – reducing the integrated person to a highly limited set of behaviours and characteristics. Making such judgements on a combination of controllable (for example, smoking) and uncontrollable (for example, family history) characteristics begins to raise questions about the use of these factors to determine health choice. It is not entirely clear to what extent access to care will be determined by 'need' or by performance against a rigid and very narrowly defined set of 'absolutes'.

The new contract requires the practice to extend health promotion activity to the wider practice population (up to the coverage targets) and particularly to people who are in a 'priority' group, again identified by the practice, for intervention. This approach, with a stronger population focus and capacity to identify and target need is consistent with the new public health approach. However, other characteristics are not. The consumer involvement in choice, the commodity approach of the first contract, is substantially reduced by the prescribed and limited content and process of the new contract. Similarly, the opportunity to promote multidisciplinary approaches is reduced by both the contraction of the field and the altered funding mechanism.

It is not clear why the emphasis on risk and risk factors has become the central plank of the new contract,[1] but the following proposals offer some thoughts. First, the 1990 arrangements were widely viewed as a 'cash cow', which enabled practices to cover the costs of a range of activities that were certainly highly attractive to patients, but were seen as of dubious or limited value by many areas of the health establishment. How such value might truly be assessed is a matter of speculation, but the result seems to have been a wish to demonstrate a 'real' outcome for the investment made, with an assumption that this would lead to health promoting or illness preventing interventions which were deemed to be appropriate and effective both for individuals and for the aggregate population.

Second, the potential challenge to professional autonomy represented by the consumer empowerment of the 1990 contract is undermined by an approach in which the first concern is risk identification, under the control of the professional within a highly defined field (CHD and stroke). This is no longer an issue of potential partnership between the patient and the doctor, but one which clearly reinforces professional sovereignty. Because there is no requirement for the GP to demonstrate that anything further than an 'offer' of health promotion has been made, there is no way to determine what level of activity and what outcome has occurred. Similarly, any challenge to medical sovereignty that may have come through the expanded and multidisciplinary activity of the 1990 contract is removed, first by contracting the range of activity, and second by removing the other professionals. As previously stated, GP fundholders' practices will have more scope to retain staff, but have also generally been far more prescriptive about the activity they wish to purchase.

DISCUSSION

While the reporting requirements aggregate risk factors across the practice within target groups, information is collated from individual profiles. With economic rationalism increasing in strength in the NHS, particularly since the introduction of the reforms, some concern might be felt that this detailed information, both individually and in aggregate, may come to be used as a basis for clinical decision making and for rationing. This may occur across all practices, fundholding or not, where either the practice itself, or the local commissioning authority, will be making decisions about the pattern of care they will purchase and in many cases about specific procedures and services. The emphasis on risk surveillance within the constraints of CHD and stroke places general practice at odds with both the multi-agency, multidisciplinary and consumer-involved approach of the new public health, but also with the main purchasers of health, the DHAs, who are working to the wider *Health of the Nation* agenda. With both sectors working towards an integrated and collaborative approach in health planning and purchasing, this mismatch may well be obstructive. If the intention of the 1993 contract included responding to the fears of GPs about increasing managerial intervention in their work, and too much 'getting into bed with the DHA', this contract creates a separate but overlapped agenda for them that permits a continued independence of approach, albeit at a high cost.

NOTES

1 It might be that, as Castel has argued, what 'the new preventive policies primarily address is no longer individuals but factors, statistical correlations of heterogeneous elements' (Castel, 1991: 288). This would suggest that emphasis on the collection of risk factors, as a tangible product, would satisfy some of the requirements for increased accountability.

Part II

Socio-political critiques of health promotion

Chapter 4

Sociological critiques of health promotion

Sarah Nettleton and Robin Bunton

INTRODUCTION

The aim of this chapter is to outline some of the existing sociological analyses and critiques of health promotion in order to identify the main parameters of the literature and to provide some pointers towards a more developed sociology of health promotion. To this end the chapter will, first, distinguish between a sociology *of* and a sociology *for* health promotion and distinguish between social and public policy approaches and sociological approaches to the analysis of health promotion. Second, it will examine three categories of sociological critique: structural, surveillance and consumption. Third, it will attempt to construct a conceptual map which relates these critiques to some key substantive areas of analysis within health promotion – populations, identities, risk and the environment.

DISCIPLINARY DISTINCTIONS AND HEALTH PROMOTION

In making sense of the literature we have found it useful to draw on two sets of distinctions which are familiar to those working within the social sciences. In Table 4.1 we have distinguished between social policy and sociological analyses of health promotion on the one hand and between analyses *of* and *for* health promotion on the other.

For those with a background in the sociology of education or medical sociology the distinction between *of* and *for* (or as applied to) is a familiar one. As long ago as the late 1950s Strauss (1957) articulated the difference between a sociology for (or in) medicine and a sociology of medicine: *for* implying that research was carried out in order to service the needs of medicine (for example, patient compliance studies), whilst a sociology *of*, by contrast, involved the study of inherently sociological concerns (for example studies examining the social basis of medical knowledge).

Thorogood (1992b) has illustrated how this distinction is particularly salient to health promotion. A sociology *for* health promotion refers to the ways in which sociology can refine and develop the techniques and practices of health promotion. The literature on lay health beliefs, for example, has illustrated the need for health promoters to take account of, and be sensitive to, the language and concepts of those audiences whom they wish to reach. It has also demonstrated that advice that is too simplistic and attempts to provide a gloss over the true complexities of illness causation is likely to be rejected (Davison *et al.*, 1992). The sociology *of* health promotion by contrast, Thorogood points out, involves a critical analysis of the underlying assumptions inherent in health promotion itself. Issues such as: the failure to reconcile the individual versus structure debate; its ideological underpinnings; the reinforcement of structural divisions and forms of discrimination; the fallacy of empowerment; and the articulation of new forms of social regulation.

Table 4.1 Social policy and sociological analyses 'for' and 'of' health promotion

	Social policy	Sociology
For	Description, analysis and evaluation of policies and policy processes, e.g. healthy public policies	Development, evaluation and refinement of promotion techniques
Of	Study of ideological basis of policies	Critiques of health promotion, e.g. structural, consumption and surveillance

The *for* and *of* distinction has also been made regarding the contribution of social policy to health promotion (Bunton, 1992a). Social policy analyses *for* refers to the ways in which the discipline can contribute to health promotion. It can provide an insight into the policy processes, potentialities and constraints which may be invaluable to those who are keen to pursue and develop healthy public policies. Clearly to promote health effectively it is necessary to understand, analyse and ultimately influence social and health policy. For example, how is it possible to create the healthy alliances espoused in *Working Together for Better Health* (Department of Health, 1993a) within the competitive environment of the internal market (Ewles, 1993)? It may also offer insights into the fate of the professionals involved in the field. For example, Lewis (1986) described the impact of the replacement of 'public health' with 'community medicine' in the 1970s and early 1980s. More recently Salter (1993) has drawn attention to the fact that the purchaser–provider split within the NHS may serve to undermine the prospects of public health doctors.

Another area pertinent to public health is the development of policies at international and global levels. For example, the extent to which Article 129 of the Maastrict Treaty is understood and interpreted could have an effect on the shape of public health and health promotion policies in the future (see Sheldon (1993)).

A social policy *of* health promotion might by contrast be more concerned to offer a critical account of the health promotion policies themselves drawing attention to their congruence with new right economic policies and the decollectivisation of welfare, such as Calnan's (1991) study of the prospects, policies and politics of preventing coronary heart disease.

As well as this *of* and *for* distinction Table 4.1 also highlights the difference between sociological and social policy approaches, especially in their analyses of the emergence of health promotion and the new public health. A social policy or socio-political explanation locates health promotion and the new public health within broader policy changes and, as we have already implied, draws attention to the fact that the rise of these disciplines fits neatly into a neo-liberal policy environment (Baggot, 1991; Mills, 1993). Such accounts can also serve to highlight the fact that they represent another arena in which there is a move towards non-collective and low-cost solutions to welfare, a deinstitutionalisation of health care, and the promotion of active citizenship.

A sociological account however is likely to have a different emphasis. It is likely to consider deeper socio-cultural shifts such as changes in the administrative technologies that deal with health problems and 'problem' populations. In recent decades the 'social' has been incorporated into these technologies. For example, epidemiology is being replaced by a more radical social epidemiology which incorporates the lay person's perspective and assumes a subjective definition of health (Scott-Samuel, 1989). Thus the changing nature of health programmes within the health promotion project serves to contribute to the construction of a new type of patient who has a different range of responsibilities. When people entered the sick role they were encouraged to interact with medical specialists – preferably doctors – whereas today, under the rubric of health promotion, people are often encouraged to actively interact with community groups, media campaigns and take responsibility for their *own* health regimes. Thus a sociological analysis of health promotion serves to demonstrate that the changing nature of these disciplines is not just the result of Government policies, but is also the effect of more fundamental discursive shifts.

Sociological critiques have in many respects contributed to the changing nature of health promotion technologies and practices. In an attempt to summarise these we have identified three broad categories: socio-structural, surveillance and consumption. We will briefly outline each of these perspectives and then consider some of the more discrete areas or issues with which each is concerned.

SOCIOLOGICAL CRITIQUES

Structural

Essentially the structural critique argues that attempts to prevent illness and to promote health have failed to take into account the material disadvantages of people's lives. This works at three levels: the political environment, the social environment and the physical environment.

Any genuine attempt to promote health must tackle the political economy that produces ill health in the first place; matters such as poverty, bad housing conditions, homelessness, poor working environments and industrial pollution. Furthermore any approach to health promotion that concentrates on telling people not to smoke rather than placing constraints on the tobacco industry must be serving the interests of capital rather than authentically pursuing good health (Doyal with Pennell, 1979). It is also inherently individualistic and behaviourist and as such results in victim blaming (Crawford, 1977; Graham, 1979; 1984).

However, health promotion has, in theory at least, overcome the limitations of this individualism. In fact by definition, it is concerned with the *twin* goals of changing both lifestyle and socio-economic-political structures (Bunton and MacDonald, 1992). Nevertheless, some critics remain unconvinced and have argued that the emphasis remains at the individual level of lifestyles. This is certainly the case at the national level as is evidenced by *The Health of the Nation*'s (Department of Health, 1992a) targets. Indeed, as McQueen (1989) has argued it is more than coincidental that the concept of health promotion emerged at a time when the dominant ideology was one of individualism. He points out that the rhetoric may be social but the actions are behaviourial and asks:

> How else can one explain a public health rhetoric which argues that social conditions affect health outcomes and then, in turn, argues that the appropriate solution is to eat better, exercise more, drink less and give up smoking?
>
> (McQueen, 1989: 342)

At a local level the emergence of the community health movement during the 1970s also attempted to counter the trends of individualism and authoritarianism (Beattie, 1991). The solution was empowerment: that is, groups of people were encouraged to take control of their own destinies, to decide amongst themselves what the most important health issues were for them, and to be supported in their attempts to bring about change (Watt, 1986). Indeed the World Health Organisation (WHO) (1985: 11) has been keen to endorse the notion that 'health developments in communities are made not only for the people but by the people'. However, critics have come to recognise the limitations of empowerment: how much power do 'community' groups really have? What kinds of changes can they realistically bring about to improve their health? To what extent do such groups become absorbed into the political structures of health care? Farrant (1991) also observes that the Government's recent interest in community development fits rather too neatly with their other aims of voluntarism, decentralisation and consumerism.

The structural critique is therefore about power. It draws attention to the fact that ideas about healthy living are promulgated by those who are white, middle class and often work within sexist, racist and homophobic value systems. This has the effect of contributing to the marginalisation of certain social groups who may be earmarked as 'targets' or 'deviant' groups (Plummer, 1988; Watney, 1988; Patton, 1990; Holland *et al.*, 1992). An example of this would be the construction of 'racial' stereotypes within the health promotion literature. Such materials may fail to acknowledge, and thereby contribute to, institutional racism, sexism and homophobia (Pearson, 1986; Thorogood, this volume).

The targeting of certain social groups or health problems may have unintended consequences for other members of society. Wang (1992) argues that prevention campaigns can have unintended and potentially negative effects. Taking the example of injury prevention campaigns in the USA she shows how the public health ethic capitalises on people's suffering. She examined responses to the two posters shown in Figure 4.1.

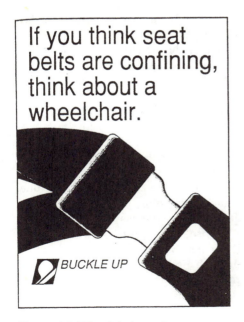

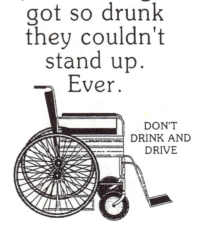

Figure 4.1 Wheelchair posters

The response of one young woman who had enrolled on a health education course to these images was:

> To me that sends a shiver, like 'God, if I was in a wheelchair'
>
> (Wang, 1992: 1089)

However, by contrast the response of a woman with a mobility disability to the same images was:

> You know, frankly, I'll look at an advertisement like this and say what's so bad about using a wheel chair. And here we go getting the message again that we're not okay as wheel chair users, or people who are blind, or use American Sign Language ... [It might be effective] for people who buy into the whole idea that disability is negative and significantly diminishes one's quality of life. Its devaluing to the rest of us who know better.
>
> (Wang, 1992: 1089)

In this respect health promotion has the potential to act as a mechanism for deviance amplification and can reinforce the stigma associated with illness or disability. It can, for example, serve to project an image of disablement as personal tragedy rather than as a socially produced state. Furthermore, it creates the sense that if illness is so bad then it must be avoided at all costs. What impact will this have on those people who are ill or especially those who have chronic conditions? There is a possibility therefore that health promotion activities can operate to create further socio-structural divisions between the 'healthy' and the 'not healthy'.

Finally, one of the most recent strands of the structural critique is that which points to the need for a green public health (Draper, 1991). This critique stresses the importance of the environment as a cause of both health and ill health. It also points to the fact that the economy and ecology are inextricably linked and that all sectors of public policy are implicated in securing safer and healthier environments. Critics speak of the political ecology of health.

Contemporary concern for a healthy environment is central to the new regime of public health. Armstrong (1993b) has outlined four regimes which have come to the fore over the last two centuries: quarantine, sanitary science, social medicine and the 'new' public health. What distinguishes the new public health is the focus on the way humans impact upon nature. Nature in itself is not a threat to health, as was the case under earlier regimes, but rather it is because of the way in which humans have spoiled nature (for example through pollution) that it has become dangerous. This argument reflects the work of Beck (1992a; 1992b) and Giddens (1990), who have both commented on the reflexive consequences of late modernity.

In short, structural critiques argue that health promotion largely fails to address the consequences of industrial capitalism: social inequalities, poverty, pollution and so on (Doyal with Pennell, 1979; Crawford, 1977; Townsend *et al.*, 1988; Draper, 1991). Further, the dominant techniques and values of health promotion and public health are congruent with capitalism in that they are elitist, individualistic and ideological (Rodmell and Watt, 1986; McQueen, 1989) as well as often being racist, sexist and homophobic (Graham, 1984; Watney, 1988; Thorogood, 1992a; Ahmad, 1993a). Consequently the reality of empowerment does not match up to the rhetoric (Beattie, 1991; Farrant, 1991).

Surveillance

What we have labelled as 'surveillance critiques' are those approaches that have focused on the programmes and technologies of health promotion and how these serve, on the one hand, to monitor and regulate populations, and, on the other hand, to construct new identities (Armstrong, 1983; Arney and Bergen, 1984; Nettleton, 1992). Contemporary health promotion techniques that aim to listen more attentively to the views of lay people, by using qualitative interviews, participant observation or health diaries, penetrate into the lives and minds of subjects. For example, dentists encourage parents and children to keep diet sheets (Nettleton, 1992: 51) and drinking diaries are often used in alcohol counselling and education (Bunton, 1990: 113). In this respect such techniques can contribute to the creation of a health promoting 'self'. One of the concerns of this critique is to alert us to the possible detrimental or constraining effects of such humanistic and liberal practices within health promotion. It suggests that whilst the sharing and exchanging of health information on more egalitarian terms might appear preferable to the didactic approaches that were characteristic of traditional health education there may still be unintended consequences. A more authoritarian health regime may be easier to challenge, ignore or reject than a supporting, caring one that sets an agenda for our lifestyles.

Another issue is the extent to which health promotion comprises programmes that result in an increasingly all-encompassing network of surveillance and observation. Armstrong (1993b) has suggested that vigilance penetrates virtually all aspects of modern life from additives in the food we eat to the state of our psyche. These observational practices are not of course restricted to health authorities but are instilled in the wider population. Health promotion techniques therefore involve more than the creation of healthy lifestyles and healthy bodies but also healthy minds and healthy subjectivities.

In fact the French philosopher Castel (1991) has suggested that we are on the verge of a medical revolution characterised by a shift from what he calls 'dangerousness to risk'. This change will see: the demise of the one-to-one practitioner–patient relationship; a new role for health professionals as health strategists; and an increasing emphasis on the profiling of populations. The target of medical care is likely to focus less on the symptoms of patients and more on their risk profile. The 'clinic of the subject', Castel argues, is being replaced by the 'epidemiological clinic' (Bunton and Burrows, this volume).

The works cited within this category have been influenced by the ideas of Foucault, especially his writings on disciplinary power. Foucault examines the ways in which forms of governance involve the investigation and regulation of the body of the individual and bodies of populations. Using a range of examples, including medicine and criminality, Foucault describes a system of surveillance which he calls *panopticism*, which has come to proliferate in modern societies. The main sites of surveillance in the nineteenth century were limited to institutions such as asylums, prisons, schools and hospitals but today the web of surveillance extends throughout the community (Armstrong, 1983). During the twentieth century the state has become increasingly important in the regulation of bodies through legislation on matters such as reproductive technologies, AIDS, childcare and so on (Turner, 1992).

In sum, within such analyses there is an emphasis on the technologies of health promotion that are seen to function as differential forms of social regulation (Arney and Bergen, 1984; Castel, 1991; Turner, 1992). It is argued that types of surveillance appear to keep expanding and changing to incorporate yet new populations and different aspects of people's lives (Bunton, 1990; Armstrong, 1993b). There is a recognition of the creation of new identities especially the 'health promoting self' – persons with an awareness of their responsibility to care for themselves (Rose, 1990; Armstrong, 1993b).

Consumption

The sociology of consumption refers to the analysis of two broad areas (Warde, 1990).[1] First, deriving from the urban sociology of Castells (1977), the study of 'consumption sector cleavages'. Such analyses are concerned with whether people *work* in the private or public sector and/or whether they *consume* predominantly from the private market or via public provision (Saunders, 1984). An example of this approach in the area of health is Calnan *et al.*'s (1993) study of the 'consumption' of private health insurance.

The second area, and one that is particularly pertinent to an analysis of health promotion, is the literature on consumer culture. This draws upon the tradition of cultural studies in order to examine consumption in relation to the construction of distinct lifestyles. Here the emphasis is often upon the consumption of goods and services which contribute to various aspects of 'body maintenance' and 'image' such as diet, sport, clothes, health clubs, etc. and is illustrated by the work of Featherstone (1991a) and Turner (1992). This links in with a developing interest in the sociology of the body (Scott and Morgan, 1993; Shilling, 1993).

The relationship between health, lifestyles and consumption is clearly a fertile ground for investigation. A key influence on this area of study is the work of Bourdieu and especially his book *Distinction* (Bourdieu, 1984). He suggests that different lifestyles are constructed as patterned assemblages of different goods (such as food, cars, furniture, clothes, body shape, sport and leisure activities) which are important markers of social difference, or distinction. This analysis draws attention to the extent to which health now forms part of lifestyles which in turn are shaped by the consumer culture in which we live. The boundaries between the health promotion literature and the commercial literature on health, lifestyles and body maintenance are increasingly blurred. Furthermore there has been what we might refer to as a decentring of health. That is, health and illness are not now confined to the clinical locations of the hospital or the GP surgery, or to relationships between doctors and patients, but are dispersed throughout various social and commercial arenas. Health promotion activities take place in a great many spheres: in our homes by way of media campaigns; in sports centres; in supermarkets; in shopping malls; at school fêtes and a whole host of other venues. Thus the distinction between the production of health and the consumption of health is collapsed. Images of health are akin to body images promulgated by the slimming, cosmetic and fitness industries (Glassner, this volume). Moreover the notion of self responsibility for health also serves the interests of both commercial entrepreneurs and health promoters.

Health education has long drawn on advertising and promotional techniques and more recently within health promotion there has been a growing emphasis on social marketing (Lefebvre, 1992). Such activities involve the symbolic communication and exchange of cultural goods. Thus the content and artefacts of health promotion lend themselves to cultural and semiotic analyses (Wang, 1992). In this respect health promoters may be regarded as members of what Bourdieu calls the 'new cultural intermediaries'. The practitioner involved in health promotion does not, as we have already suggested, engage in one-to-one relationships, but is party to the creation and marketisation of a certain way of living. Health promotion therefore is central to the creation of what Wernick (1991) has recently termed 'a promotional culture'.

In summary, analyses of health promotion drawing upon the sociology of consumption emphasise the extent to which health promotion involves cultural processes (Farrant and Russell, 1986; Bunton *et al.*, 1991; Wang, 1992; Lupton, 1994). They also focus on the structuring of 'choice' and the construction of identities through health promotion practices and the commodification of health products (Featherstone, 1991a; Grace, 1991). Such approaches are also interested in the way in which the products of health promoters – such as fitness programmes and diets – are 'aestheti- sized' under consumer culture and may become a means of communi- cation of status and group identity (Glassner, 1989).

THE SOCIOLOGY OF HEALTH PROMOTION: TOWARDS A CONCEPTUAL MAP

Having outlined three categories of sociological critique it is now possible to identify and map them out in relation to some key substantive concerns or foci of health promotion activity, as shown in Table 4.2. We have selected four broad topics all of which are both central to the activities of health promotion and are evident within all three critiques. Health promotion activity is, for the most part, directed at promoting the health of *populations*. However, at the same time, such activities serve to contrib- ute to the creation of individual *identities*. Both populations and indi- viduals are envisaged in terms of differential *risk* factors. Indeed the reduction of risk, in many respects, could be said to be the very stuff of health promotion. Such risk reduction requires that adequate attention be paid to the *environmental* context in which people live out their lives. We do not claim to offer an exhaustive typology, however we suggest that the following provides a useful initial conceptual map of the terrain to be covered by an adequate sociology of health promotion. The rest of the chapter will briefly elaborate upon the contents of each cell in Table 4.2 and, where possible, locate some of the existing sociological literature.

Table 4.2 Critiques of health promotion and the foci of health promotion

| Critiques | Foci of health promotion | | | |
	Populations	Identities	Risk	Environment
Structural	Control of 'problem' groups	Victim blaming	Material circumstances	Politics of pollution
Surveillance	Technologies e.g. surveys, diaries	Health promoting self	Rational calculation/ probabilities	Human-made environmental dangers
Consumption	Social marketing	Consuming healthy lifestyles/ images	Buying security e.g. Volvos, extra virgin olive oil	Greening of commercial products

Taking first the structural critique, the *structural/population* cell refers to those activities that reinforce social divisions and thereby contribute to class divisions, sexism, racism and homophobia. This is because health promotion programmes often attempt to control the behaviours of certain 'problem' groups through the promulgation and legitimation of dominant norms and values. The lifestyles of social groups may be 'targeted' for alteration by health promoters. This can, according to the structural critique, have the effect of pathologising health problems within the selected social groups and, at the same time, affirming the health beliefs and behaviours of structurally advantaged social groups. Certainly some AIDS health promotion activities, especially those based on the information-giving model, have contributed to and reinforced homophobia and discriminatory practices (Watney, 1988; Patton, 1990). For example, some critics have taken health promoters to task for speaking about 'risk groups' rather than 'risk behaviours'. This reinforces 'the dubious idea that it is risk group susceptibilities rather than how one engages in specific sexual and drug acts that creates the possibility of HIV transmission' (Patton, 1990: 103). Similarly some health education programmes directed at 'ethnic minorities', campaigns such as those concerned with rickets, surma and antenatal care, have contributed to the construction of racist stereotypes, and as such augment institutional racism (Pearson, 1986) rather than addressing more appropriate health needs.

There is also an irony here. Whilst health promotion is often targeted at those who are structurally disadvantaged it is those who are in structurally advantaged positions who benefit most from the changes in lifestyle advocated by health promoters. Evidence suggests that changes in individual health behaviours do not have a uniform impact upon the population. For those in structurally disadvantaged social positions individual behavioural change has relatively little impact upon health status. However, for those in structurally advantaged positions the causal efficacy of individual behavioural change can be important. As Blaxter concludes from her study of *Health and Lifestyles*, '[o]nly in the more favourable circumstances is there "room" for considerable damage or improvement by the adoption of voluntary health-related habits' (Blaxter, 1990: 223). Thus, health promotion may contribute to the exacerbation of existing health inequalities. Despite this observation the vast majority of research into health-related behaviours has focused on the structurally disadvantaged with only a few studies giving any explicit sociological attention to the health-related habits of structurally advantaged social groups (Calnan, 1987; Backett, 1992; Burrows and Nettleton, 1995).

An effect of the evaluations of populations might be the creation of negative self-images and victim blaming which is located in the *structural/ identities* cell. Perhaps the classic example here is that of 'guilty' mothers who have long been the traditional target of health education. Whilst the discourse of health promotion emphasises the merits of providing people with knowledge and information so that they can make healthy choices, the structural critique suggests that the notion of individual choice is a mythical one and draws attention to the fact that health promotion makes people feel responsible and culpable for their health status. This has become evident in a number of areas, for example Graham's (1987) research on women and smoking, Nettleton's (1986) work on mothers and their children's dental health and Davison *et al*.'s (1992) studies of heart disease during the Heartbeat Wales Campaign.

Within the *structural/risks* cell, health risks are identified as being predominantly associated with structural disadvantage and people's material circumstances such as poverty, bad housing, poor working conditions and polluted environments. It is these factors that raise the likelihood of accidents, death and illness (Doyal with Pennell, 1979). Such structural explanations are thus critical of approaches that focus on more behavioural factors especially the holy trinity of risks: smoking, exercise and diet (Martin and McQueen, 1989; Davey Smith *et al*., 1990).

The *structural/environment* cell contains those critiques that concern the environment highlighting the relationship between capitalism and pollution (Draper, 1991). Hunt's (1989) work on private cars illustrates this well. As she points out, the health effects of cars (pollution, accidents, etc.) are significant in comparison to other health risks such as exercise. Yet the health effects of private cars have largely escaped serious attention. This is because people with cars tend to regard them as essential for their lifestyles, the road lobby is so politically powerful and cars are a significant source of tax revenue. Health promotion associated with private cars, Hunt argues, should not just be limited to drink drive campaigns and educating people to be safe drivers but must also address more fundamental environmental policies such as urban design and the development of comprehensive transport policies. Public transport systems can be designed to reduce pollution and engender regular exercise through the provision of cycle tracks, walkways and easily accessible city transport. Such systems would avoid many of the environmental and health ill-effects of those which currently privilege the motor car (Hillman, 1991).

Populations are the most readily obvious focus of the surveillance critique. The *surveillance/population* cell includes the identification and evaluation of the technologies of monitoring, assessing, profiling and developing population-based interventions. These measures can result in legally unprecedented incursions into people's lives and threats to previously defined civil liberties (Gostin, 1986). Plummer (1988) illustrates this when he articulates concern about the monitoring of the sexual activities of gay people:

> with the symbolism of AIDS has emerged a range of institutional practices that aim to increase surveillance and regulation over 'deviances' and 'sexualities', many new agencies have appeared along with

many new practices that aim to keep records, classify and order, take tests, watch over, maybe brand and quarantine people on the AIDS spectrum ... Small trends can become big institutions; what has emerged in the past few years may very well proliferate and extend ... establishing firm new structures for the control of 'deviance' and 'sexuality' by the end of the century.

(Plummer, 1988: 46)

Similar concerns have been noted in relation to the monitoring of illicit drug taking in the workplace and other public settings (Bakalar and Grinspoon, 1984).

An effect of the technologies associated with the surveillance of populations is the construction of individual selves and especially the social construction of the health promoting self – this is the focus of *surveillance/identity* cell. As people become caught within the discourses of health promotion they become increasingly aware of the contributions that they themselves can make to the project of health maintenance and this may in turn impact upon how they reflect upon, monitor and think about themselves. The vocabulary of health promoters and 'experts' provides one of the multiplicity of discourses that lay people may draw upon to interpret their own experiences and construct them*selves*. For example, in a study of dental health education Nettleton (1991) found how the language of dental health educators came to be shared by mothers who are variously constructed as 'natural', 'ignorant', 'responsible' and 'caring'. According to Rose (1990) even our own private thoughts are created and shaped by social institutions, education, and activities derived from the social sciences; in other words, the 'technologies of the self', of which health promotion programmes would be but one example. These are 'the ways in which we are enabled, by means of the languages, criteria, and techniques offered to us, to act upon our bodies, souls, thoughts and conduct in order to achieve happiness, wisdom, health and fulfilment' (Rose, 1990: 10). Thus from this perspective, health promotion can be seen as one of many forms of contemporary governance which, through the establishment of appropriate social identities forms a crucial dimension of effective social regulation. This idea resonates with some of the recent writings of Giddens (1991; 1992) who has begun to explore the forms of subjectivity that are emerging in response to late modernism. His conceptualisation contends that the defining characteristic of contemporary self-identity is its *reflexivity*: the idea that most aspects of social life can be subject to strategic transformation and modification on the basis of new knowledge and the capacity to discursively interpret conduct.

The *surveillance/risk* cell alludes to the way in which health 'risks' are derived from aggregate level data and are based on probabilities which, in turn, can be monitored. Personal risks, for example a child having an accident, become systematic events which then require political regulation (Green, this volume; Prior, this volume). Seemingly personal choices and activities such as eating cream cakes become absorbed into systematic risks which are then amenable to monitoring and regulation. Further, accidents and illnesses that appear to be, at first sight, highly personal in their consequences are at the same time 'systematically caused, statistically describable and in that sense "predictable" types of events'. It means that everyone is subject to 'political rules of recognition, compensation and avoidance' (Beck, 1992b: 99). This is what, as we have seen, Castel refers to as the 'epidemiological clinic': the creation of the category of risk has come to serve as a technique of governance.

Within the *surveillance/environment* cell threats to health are those that fall beyond the boundaries of calculable risk. Although not writing about health promotion as such Beck (1992a; 1992b) and Giddens (1990) have drawn attention to the unimaginable and potentially devastating consequences of the 'person made environment', for example the threat of nuclear fallout, modern warfare and genetic engineering. Whilst misfortunes in preindustrial societies were attributable to fate, God(s) or natural disasters, modern risks are increasingly created by the social and economic processes associated with industrialisation. They argue that modernity both produces risks (through working conditions, means of transport, pollution and the like) and, as we have discussed above, compensates for them by means of calculation and political regulation. However, the calculations of risk are becoming increasingly difficult, if not impossible, because of the emergence of phenomena which have unimaginable consequences – 'nuclear, chemical, genetic and ecological mega-hazards abolish the ... calculus of risks' (Beck, 1992b: 101–2). They are global in scope, there is no satisfactory aftercare following their activation, and there are no statistical bases for their calculation. This growing sensitivity to risk also results in a heightened level of anxiety which, as we have already noted, is further exacerbated by a decline in the faith of 'experts' (Giddens, 1990: 130; Beck, 1992b).

Writing more specifically on public health issues, Williams and Popay (1994) illustrate how these trends are evidenced in the case of the Camelford poisoning episode in Cornwall. In 1988 a lorry driver accidentally tipped 20 tonnes of aluminium sulphate solution into a treated water reservoir. Williams and Popay describe the actions taken by the local residents who were not prepared to passively accept the findings of the 'expert' committee of inquiry into the affair. The balance between lay and professional knowledge may well be shifting and this may be enhanced by the uncertain and incalculable nature of environmental risks associated with late modernity. As Williams and Popay (1994: 120) point out, examples such as the Camelford case represent both an *epistemological* challenge to expert knowledge and a *political* 'challenge to the institutional power of expert knowledge in general, and medical knowledge in particular'.

Whilst the sociology of consumption in relation to health promotion is less developed than the other two categories discussed above, we can nevertheless begin to identify distinct areas of study. The *consumption/ populations* cell might focus on the congruence of health promotion and marketing techniques and health promotion's complicity with broader consumer (Bunton and Burrows, this volume; Glassner, this volume) and promotional culture (Wernick, 1991). This is illustrated by the growing use by health promoters of increasingly sophisticated marketing techniques which were inititated and developed within the commercial sector (O'Brien, 1992; this volume). As we have discussed above, these techniques of 'social marketing' within health promotion are 'programmes . . . developed to satisfy consumers needs, strategised to reach the audience(s) in need of the programme, and managed to meet organisational objectives' (Lefebvre, 1992: 153). Conversely, the commercial sector during the last decade has increasingly drawn on the language and rhetoric of health promoters. For example, a current advertisement for Kellogg's Bran Flakes suggests that their consumption provides an easy route into adopting a healthy lifestyle. A man clad in his dressing gown eats his bran flakes whilst watching an exercise video. His arm movements work in time with the exercises. The implication is that this is as much exercise as he is ever likely to get around to. In this respect the advertisers draw on a tension which is inherent in health promotion: that healthy living is both good for you and fun and yet at the same time it is laborious and dull.

In this respect, unlike the marketing of commercial products the social marketing of health promotion is faced by a dilemma. It is likely that promotional activities are most effective if they tap into a corpus of existing meanings, rather than attempting to create new ones. Most successful marketing appropriates desired abstract values such as glamour, vitality, sensuality, youthfulness and so on as 'floating signifiers' which are then used to give meaning to otherwise meaningless products (Featherstone, 1991b: 174). Ironically, whilst such signifiers appear to be relatively easy to 'fix' to products not considered to be 'really healthy' (Mars Bars, Coca-Cola, Pepsi, Lucozade, lager, cosmetics and so on) they are not so easy to attach to products which are (vegetables, seat-belts, condoms and so on).

The marketing of health by both commercial and non-commercial organisations is about the creation of wants, needs and desires. Grace (1991) in a study of health promoters working in community development in New Zealand found that there were direct parallels between the discourse of empowerment and the discourse of marketing. People are encouraged to find ways of meeting their self-defined needs. However these needs, Grace points out, are frequently set by a pre-given agenda. Indeed the very process of the identification of needs itself serves to construct people as 'consumers' who have a need and desire for health status. She says: 'Health promotion, rather than fulfilling its promise of empowerment, effectively constructs the individual as a 'health consumer' in accordance with the model of consumer capitalism' (Grace, 1991: 330).

The *consumption/identities* cell alludes to the ways in which personal and group identities are engendered through the consumption of commodities – from health magazines to health farms. Glassner's (1989) account of fitness and the development of the postmodern self provides a good example of this process. Health promotion is symptomatic of wider cultural change involving the fabrication of more reflexive late modern self-identities. This in turn demands of the self and the body a greater 'plasticity' which can only be achieved by the subtle calculation of appropriate patterns of consumption akin to those expounded by health promotion. Contemporary self-identities are largely constituted through role-playing, image construction and the consumption of goods and services with varying identity-values located in the spheres of culture, leisure, play and consumption (Kellner, 1992). The ubiquity of images of 'health' and 'healthy living' in these domains are thus important sources of contemporary self-identity. However, these images of health are strongly mediated by other cultural sources of self-identity which emphasise the glamour, danger, toughness, rebelliousness and sexuality associated with the consumption of unhealthy products such as tobacco and alcohol (Amos, 1992).

The *consumption/risk* cell refers to the encouragement to think about the consumption of things in terms of risk. There is a sense in which people may 'buy into security', for example, choosing extra virgin olive oil to reduce the risk of heart disease or buying a Volvo car because of its association with safety. Indeed, the discourse of health promotion encourages the subtle calculation of a calculus of risk in almost everything we consume (three egg-sized potatoes a day, three-quarters of a bar of chocolate a week, 21 units of alcohol a week . . .). However, whilst health promotion encourages a culture of risk minimisation, many commodities are consumed precisely because they are associated with high levels of risk and, within certain cultural settings, are attractive for this very reason (drugs, motorbikes, fast cars and so on). 'Risk-takers' as an identity category (Plant and Plant, 1992) provides an interesting conceptual link between this cell and the previous cell.

The *consumption/environment* cell refers to analyses of consumption practices at the interface of health promotion and environmental politics. The marrying of ecological concerns with the new public health forms the central plank of the 'healthy cities' agenda (Davies and Kelly, 1993). The articulation of green 'eco' sound products with the imagery of healthy lifestyles more generally has become a feature of much recent product development and marketing. The 'greening' of consumer culture over the last decade has corresponded with, and is clearly linked to, the emergence of the discourse of health promotion.

CONCLUSION

This chapter provided a review of sociological analyses *of* health promotion and grouped these into three approaches or forms of critique: structural, surveillance and consumption. These approaches were then developed in relation to four key foci of health promotion, namely populations, identities, risk and the environment. The intention has been to provide a conceptual map of the existing literature in the hope that it may provide a basis for debate and further research. In this respect a number of observations can be made.

First, the literature within the structural critique appears to be more prolific and well developed in comparison to that within the surveillance and consumption critiques. This is perhaps hardly surprising given it has the longest history. Indeed, there is a chronology to these analyses with the consumption critique being the most recent to be applied to health promotion and the least researched. Given the congruity between health promotion activities and the commercialisation of health-related goods, services and activities, empirical accounts of consumption practices would seem to be of particular relevance to both theoretical analyses and to the activities of health promotion.

Second, with few exceptions (Rawson and Grigg, 1988), there has been little published research into the institutional and professional developments of either health promotion or the new public health. In fact such studies are noticeable by their absence. This is surprising given the significance of research within the sociology of health and illness into processes of professionalisation and the nature of professional knowledge. Certainly these have been extensively explored in relation to other areas of medical and paramedical practice. Sociological analyses of health promotion have tended to focus on those areas which are of concern to the practitioners themselves, thereby focusing on the recipients of, rather than the peddlers of, health promotion. What remains relatively unexplored are the perceptions, activities and knowledge base of those working within those institutions concerned with the delivery of health promotion programmes and policies. In other words a sociology of professional (health promotion) knowledge.

Third, much of the current concerns of contemporary sociological theory appears to be particularly significant to the analysis of health promotion. They are concerned with matters such as risk, identity and the environment. Furthermore the health promotion project itself is in many respects characteristic of late modernism. It is imperative therefore that sociological analysts of health promotion, and health promoters who wish to draw upon sociology to develop their practice, move beyond structural approaches and try to integrate, by way of both empirical and theoretical research, more recent developments within sociology.

NOTES

1 A third area of interest might be the distribution of goods consumed within households (for example Charles and Kerr's (1988) study of the distribution of food within households). Although often not thought of as being part of the sociology of consumption, feminist analyses of food, smoking, car use, etc. can be conceptualised in this way. Clearly, this literature overlaps with the structural critique with which we have already dealt.

Chapter 5

Feminist critiques of health promotion

Norma Daykin and Jennie Naidoo

INTRODUCTION

Health promotion is a hybrid activity. The broad aims of health promotion are not easily distinguished from other health care goals. However, in the UK health promotion is identified in the main as a specialised form of provision oriented towards the primary and secondary prevention of specific conditions such as coronary heart disease and cancers. The recently published Government strategy for health promotion, *The Health of the Nation* (Department of Health, 1992a), has prioritised and legitimised this approach. These characteristics influence the organisational framework for the delivery of health promotion within the NHS. Whether this takes place in health promotion departments or within primary health care, Government targets are increasingly important.

Feminist activists have been involved in health promotion at many levels and in different ways. Given the different varieties of health promotion and of feminism, there can be no simple, universal feminist critique of health promotion. In this chapter, we shall examine a range of perspectives, drawing on feminist critiques of medicine to identify ways in which sexism has influenced the design and delivery of health promotion. For example, the neglect of women's experience of morbidity and mortality has led to the development of targets based on male-centred epidemiology. When women's health problems are identified in health promotion, these tend to be medicalised leading at times to inappropriate and ineffective solutions. In addition, health promotion strategies may place responsibility for health on women without recognising their relative lack of power to effect change. The victim blaming that results from conventional health promotion approaches impacts upon women as carers, by ignoring the socio-economic context and social marginalisation of that caring role.

Feminist critiques of health promotion have many sources of inspiration to draw upon, most notably traditions of political activism and the women's health movement. These movements have sought to contextualise women's health within a socio-economic environment, and to identify strategies that enable a collective response. There is a need to develop policies and services which are accessible, appropriate, and enhance the ability of women to resist the health-eroding pressures of their daily lives.

For the sake of clarity, we shall adopt Beattie's framework for analysing health promotion (Beattie, 1991). This framework identifies health promotion activities around the dimensions of authoritative/negotiated and individual/collective, and is summarised in Figure 5.1. However, it should be borne in mind that these are models and that practice rarely fits a single one. The most effective women-centred health promotion would utilise more than one 'type', as well as forms of practice which do not easily lend themselves to such categorisation.

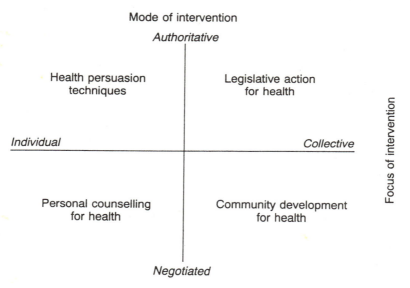

Figure 5.1 Models of health promotion
Source: Beattie (1991)

INDIVIDUALLY FOCUSED HEALTH PROMOTION

Beattie (1991) characterises this kind of health promotion as being focused on the individual, either controlled in an authoritarian manner by people who claim expert status, or negotiated using techniques such as education and counselling. Much traditional health education takes place in this way, based on a philosophy reemphasised in the 1970s, that the responsibility for ensuring good health rests with the individual (DHSS, 1976a).

Individually focused health promotion has been criticised for failing to take into account the structural constraints on people's lives. For example, Oakley (1989) has argued that conventional smoking cessation campaigns aimed at women are based on a theoretical model in which smoking is seen as an irrational form of behaviour. Health education within this model seeks to make good the deficits in women's beliefs and knowledge through information campaigns. However, women demonstrate high levels of awareness about current medical evidence relating smoking to health outcomes. This awareness did not influence the behaviour of the women in Oakley's study, which was instead related to the deeper patterns of class and gender division which shaped their lives. Women who experienced low levels of social support and poor material conditions during pregnancy were particularly likely to smoke.

Similarly, Graham (1987) found that for women caring for children on a low income, smoking offered a means of coping. Cigarettes helped by creating a structure for the day, providing a break and allowing both physical and emotional distance from children in situations where there was no alternative outlet or escape. Women's smoking behaviour was reinforced by patterns of living in low-income households where women retain responsibility for budgeting without the power to determine outcomes for their families. Whilst budgeting, along with caring, represents an important dimension of health promotion within households, spending on tobacco was demonstrated as the exception to the rule by which fixed costs and collective costs are met first. In both of these accounts, a complex relationship between smoking, caring and material disadvantage was seen as leading to the paradoxical rule that 'health promoting work may be damaging for those who do it' (Oakley, 1989: 329).

Campaigns that aim to achieve individual behavioural change simply through persuasion are therefore flawed and may even be counterproductive. This is because such campaigns construct behaviour such as smoking as a lifestyle choice, rather than understanding it within a material and cultural framework incorporating an analysis of class, gender and other inequalities. Critics of the individual approach have highlighted the limitations of the 'lifestyle-choice' model in which people are seen as consumers exercising market choice between healthy and unhealthy products (Naidoo, 1986). Women, particularly those on low incomes and in marginalised employment, do not easily fit the stereotype of an independent consumer. They are likely to be alienated from health promotion campaigns which rely on an appeal to such a constituency, as is to some extent demonstrated in the research finding that members of low income groups tend to make the least use of preventive medicine and health education despite experiencing the poorest health (Townsend *et al.*, 1988).

The increased use of market analogies in health and welfare in recent years has reinforced the 'lifestyle-choice' model, which offers most to those with the economic and political resources with which to exercise meaningful choices. At the same time, inequalities in society have widened, as a result of increased unemployment and 'flexible' working patterns including casual, part-time and low-paid employment (Brown and Scase, 1991). This has led to the increased marginalisation of some groups, especially poor single mothers, for whom deprivation is increasingly recognised as a critical influence on health-related behaviour (Marsh and McKay, 1994; Phillimore *et al.*, 1994).

Whilst some critics see individually focused health advice as a limited but useful part of a wider strategy, others have argued that such strategies, by adopting a 'victim-blaming' approach, can serve as a distraction from the real issues. Kenner (1985) points out that since society is not organised around health as a priority, women often find themselves unable to make healthy choices, because the choices most readily available represent unhealthy options. For example, low-cost council housing may be inadequately insulated, damp, or have design features which compromise safety.

However, the role of advice, information giving and counselling, in both one-to-one and group settings, has been central to the development of the women's health movement. In this example individually focused strategies are integrated within an approach that also recognises the collective nature of many women's health issues. Personal space and time to identify and share health experiences has had a cumulative and significant effect, in that many women's health problems are no longer shrouded in secrecy. Hence whilst feminist health activism may make good use of individually focused strategies, the model of the individual as consumer is inappropriate for many women.

Current policies, such as the GP banding payments for health promotion, are individually focused, encouraging opportunistic, one-to-one health education during routine consultations. This form of health promotion may indeed form a useful part of a wider strategy. Research has shown that general practitioners are seen as a credible source of information on smoking, for example, and that many women take action following advice from a doctor or other member of the practice staff (Blackburn and Graham, 1993). Counselling and other techniques such as assertiveness training may also be useful interventions, for example in the field of sexual health and HIV/AIDS prevention. These techniques are likely to appeal to health professionals who wish to work in supportive, non-authoritarian ways. Whether authoritative or negotiated, individually focused health promotion needs to be backed up with strategies that address broader issues. Telling women not to smoke without examining the pressures that lead to the desire for a cigarette is problematic, in the same way as is counselling women to adopt safer sexual practices without recognising the unequal power relationships that construct sexuality, or challenging the cultural privilege afforded to penetrative hetero-sexual sex (Lees, 1986; Wilton, 1994).

Whilst women are often constrained from exercising consumer choice in their own right, they are frequently targeted as carers in conventional health promotion campaigns. These assume women's responsibility for the health of others. At worst, this assumption leads to the use of images such as the one used by the Health Education Council during the 1980s featuring a pregnant woman and a warning about the effects of smoking on the unborn child. Strongly criticised by feminists, this campaign gave a clear message about women's responsibilities for the health of others, with the implication that the effects of smoking on women themselves are less worthy of consideration. This message also ignores the effects of male smoking behaviour on the health of children and women.

On a more general level, women are assumed to be responsible for health promotion within the family, through the inculcation of healthy lifestyles and the provision of informal health care for children, spouses and other relatives (Graham, 1984; 1988). This responsibility extends from maintaining and protecting family health through everyday activities such as cleaning, washing and cooking, through to the 'emotional housework' of dealing with the stresses experienced by individual family members (Doyal, 1991). In addition, women are often expected to act as mediators between households and health services, by, for example, deciding when family members need to visit the doctor, and accompanying or making arrangements for such visits. Even when women are not directly providing such services, the responsibility for ensuring that such needs are met on a daily basis falls on their shoulders.

Assumptions of women's roles affect both informal and more formal health promotion activities. For example, nutrition campaigns are often targeted at women in their role of food provider for families. However, this may trigger conflicts for women, who end up balancing health edu-cation messages with other priorities, such as providing food which is familiar and liked by other family members, and buying food within tightly constrained budgets (Charles and Kerr, 1986). It has been demon-strated that providing a healthy diet is beyond the means of many women on low incomes (Cole-Hamilton, 1987), and that household priorities dictate that women and children eat lower status foods than men (Charles and Kerr, 1987). All too often, the impact of health education campaigns has been to make women feel guilty because they cannot respond posi-tively to the health education message. This is because such campaigns confer responsibility on women without recognising the powerlessness that underlies their health promoting work. The overall outcome may then be increased stress and ill health for women (Doyal, 1995).

It can be seen then that the paradox of 'responsibility without power' underpins many health promotion activities that are directed at women.

On a broader level, feminist critiques have challenged social policy discourses which construct women as carers, thus naturalising gender inequalities. Informal health promotion activities are assumed to belong to women because of their 'caring' nature, an assumption reflected in community care policies which reinforce women's role as informal carers (Baldwin and Twigg, 1991; Finch, 1984). This role is further enshrined in labour market structures that lead to the concentration of women in part-time employment, resulting in lower pay, reduced rights and reduced opportunities for training and promotion (Charles, 1993).

This is not to deny that many women choose to care as a fulfilling and meaningful experience. Conventional feminist accounts of caring have been challenged in recent writings, such as work by bell hooks on the impact of slavery and racism on the construction of the African-American homeplace. In this context the decision to care is seen as a positive, political and humanising response to oppressive forces that devalue black family life (bell hooks, 1991). Disabled women have further broadened this debate, arguing that by focusing attention on the needs of unpaid carers, feminists have contributed to the assumption that disabled people represent a 'problem' for society, undermining the rights of disabled women to self-determination and independence (Morris, 1993).

These interpretations should lead not to the abandonment of critiques of care, but to a recognition of the need to value women's caring as work. By constructing such care as a natural attribute of womanhood, the possibilities for providing support for this activity are reduced. This is the logic behind many government policies which have constructed what has been called women's 'compulsory altruism' (Land and Rose, 1985). The result is to erode the rights, and the health, of women and of those about whom they care.

COLLECTIVELY FOCUSED HEALTH PROMOTION

This kind of health promotion is directed towards communities, and includes both authoritative and negotiated approaches (Beattie, 1991). The former includes services such as immunisation and screening, currently linked in the UK to Government targets, which represent a medicalised type of provision. Collective authoritarian approaches may also reflect a social model of health, encompassing broader social policy initiatives ranging from tobacco control to housing provision. In both cases, authority remains with experts such as doctors and policy makers who are seen as having specialist knowledge.

In the UK, the medical model has tended to dominate health service provision, including health promotion. For example, the targets identified in *The Health of the Nation* (Department of Health, 1992a) are derived from a top-down assessment of public health priorities. These targets aim to reduce death rates in key areas such as coronary heart disease, strokes and cancers, as well as bringing about improvements in areas such as sexual health. Whilst these health issues affect many women, feminist perspectives have highlighted ways in which the targets are constructed around male health patterns. For example, the targets focus on premature mortality, ignoring conditions such as arthritis and osteoporosis, which contribute to women's excess morbidity (Roberts, 1990; Miles, 1991). Diseases such as lung cancer and coronary heart disease are important causes of death amongst women (Miles, 1991; Wells, 1987). However, these are still often constructed as 'male' problems and preventive strategies may be based on findings from research that fails to take into account the impact of sex differences in causes and treatment outcomes (Doyal, 1995).

Hence sexism in medical research and epidemiology has led to the setting of public health priorities, and the development of services, based on the experience of men. In addition, women's health problems tend to be medicalised. Thus women's cancers are prioritised within the context of national screening programmes which are not of proven effectiveness (Thompson and Brown, 1990; Skrabanek, 1988; Schwartz et al., 1989). Similarly, the menopause is constructed as a biological deficit treatable by hormone replacement therapy (Miles, 1991).

When women are targeted by collectively focused health promotion initiatives it is again often in their assumed role as carers, and their responsibility for promoting the health of others is taken for granted. Mothers are targeted more than fathers in child immunisation campaigns, for example, which may add to the burden of guilt. Women are more likely therefore to come into contact with medicalised forms of health promotion, not only through the experience of pregnancy and childbirth (Oakley, 1984), but throughout their careers as carers.

Feminists have been concerned to document the impact of the medicalisation of health care on women, and the ways in which medicalisation interacts with gender inequalities (Doyal, 1994). The *Health of the Nation* strategy relies on a combination of screening and health persuasion, with resources targeted towards primary health care. However, the primary health care setting is not gender neutral. Although women now constitute 50 per cent of student doctors, only 20 per cent of GPs are female (NHS Management Executive, 1992). The medical model still assumes a dominant professional and a passive patient, and overlaid on this pattern is the stereotype of the male doctor and the female patient.

Feminist accounts of medicine have sought to highlight male bias in the medical profession both in terms of ideology and practice. The conflation of notions of masculinity and expertise has been seen as increasing male control over women, who are pathologised as inherently unhealthy, either sick or sickening (Broverman et al., 1970; Ehrenreich and English,

1973). By endorsing what is commonly accepted as normal, natural and healthy for women, health promoters are seen as contributing towards the social construction of femininity around the requirements of the heterosexual monogamous nuclear family (Smart, 1992). In some accounts of 1970s radical feminism, screening and health promotion were viewed with suspicion as an extension of medical control, part of a regulatory machinery enforcing male notions of femininity 'typified by the weak, "normal" woman whose normality is so elusive that it must constantly be reinforced through regular check-ups, "preventative medicine" and perpetual therapy' (Daly, 1979: 231).

Medical control does not impact uniformly on all women. Whilst the activities which Daly describes are more likely to involve women from higher income groups, the more punitive aspects of medicalised forms of social control impact disproportionately on disadvantaged groups. Feminists have documented how black women are more likely to be offered sterilisation and more dangerous forms of contraception than are white women (Amos and Parmar, 1984; Bryan *et al.*, 1985; Anthias and Yuval-Davis, 1983).

An account that views medicine purely as a form of social control underplays the benefits to women of contemporary health care. In the current climate of health care rationing, feminist activists are more concerned that screening does not reach the women who are most at risk from diseases such as cancer of the cervix, where early detection can make a significant difference to treatment outcomes. National screening programmes, whilst not unquestionably successful, have served to put diseases such as breast cancer on the agenda, thereby reducing the secrecy and fear that may inhibit women from seeking treatment. Black women have been active in lobbying for a national sickle cell screening, counselling and information programme (Prashar, *et al.*, 1985), arguing that a lack of such facilities increases misdiagnosis, illness and avoidable deaths.

Nevertheless the trend towards analysing and monitoring populations has been seen as leading to increased social regulation, surveillance of the 'well' in addition to the sick through the notion of 'risk' (Bunton, 1992b). Sex education has also been defined in this way, with its focus on the body, constructed through notions of heterosexual desire, providing scope for increased interventions (Thorogood, 1992a).

The social construction of gender and sexuality has influenced the design and delivery of health promotion in the field of HIV/AIDS prevention. Educational materials on safer sex for women are scarcer, and less explicit than those available to men (Wilton, 1994). Yet women are targeted in some health promotion campaigns when their HIV status is seen as providing general information (as in the anonymous screening of women at antenatal clinics), or when their sexual behaviour is assumed to represent a threat to men. Women sex workers are often viewed as a vector of infection, endangering men and the 'general population', despite evidence which suggests that it is male clients who demand unprotected sex, and that it is easier for men to infect women during sexual intercourse than vice versa (Bury, 1994).

The impact of different preoccupations concerning gender and sexuality may result in state organisations working at odds with each other. For example, the *Health of the Nation* strategy includes a reduction in the rate of teenage pregnancy which is targeted at young women (Department of Health, 1992a). However, simultaneous moves to devolve to a local level the responsibility for sex education in schools, which effectively fragments and restricts sex education, make this target more difficult to reach.

This example demonstrates the importance of replacing such contradictory policies with an integrated approach where collective strategies are reinforced by broader social policies to promote health. To take the case of tobacco control, the Government has favoured price control through increased taxation as a means of reducing smoking rates in the population. Whilst this measure may be effective for the majority, research has shown that a significant group of poor smokers are impervious to price increases, making tobacco taxation one of the most regressive forms of taxation in the UK, and resulting in real hardship for many low-income households (Marsh and McKay, 1994). At the same time, the Government is reluctant to adopt what it sees as an authoritarian stance towards the producers and promoters of tobacco, which it is argued would lead to lower smoking rates especially amongst young people (Mindell, 1992). Instead, the Government has favoured voluntary agreements and self regulation in tobacco advertising. Feminists have been amongst the critics of these voluntaristic policies, which are seen as piecemeal and ineffective (Jacobson, 1986). Feminist campaigners are keen to develop collective policies that address the connections between low income, caring, tobacco control, and smoking without further penalising poor women (Action on Smoking and Health (ASH) Women and Smoking Group, 1993).

Other forms of collective provision may be negotiated, drawing on a community development approach which emphasises outreach work, and addresses the concerns of users even though these may not correspond to medically defined priorities. Community development, with its focus on the collective and social nature of health, its explicit attempt to reduce inequalities in health, and its emphasis on the process of empowerment, does not produce easily quantifiable outcomes. As a result, it is difficult to secure funding for such initiatives, which tend to be marginalised, surviving on a local basis as a result of piecemeal resourcing from a variety of agencies.

Whilst the effectiveness of community development approaches may be difficult to demonstrate in the short term, the effectiveness of current approaches based on routine health checks and advice is increasingly called into question (Stott, 1994). Community-based initiatives, backed up with effective legislation to regulate harmful products, may represent a useful alternative to primary health care workers who are increasingly cynical about existing strategies. In the current climate it is difficult to see how community development approaches fit in with health promotion in primary health care. However, imaginative interpretation of GP contract and banding arrangements could provide an impetus for working with a range of groups and organisations. Hence with support and encouragement, primary health care workers could draw on the expertise that exists within the women's health movement, at the same time as fulfilling the requirements of current policies. Community consultation may for example result in increased take-up of screening and may also reduce costs incurred by unnecessary prescribing.

Much of the activity generated by community development activities focuses on women and their health concerns. Hence community development has been acclaimed as a strategy which enables feminist health promotion (Rodmell and Watt, 1986). Accounts of community development health projects often stress the real impact made on women's lives, and emphasise the increase in women's knowledge, skills and self-esteem which result (Aird, 1986; Research Unit in Health and Behaviour Change, 1989; Roberts, 1992). Community development may also be viewed as a strategy which can professionalise 'feminine' skills such as networking, sharing and supporting.

This approach does however carry the risk of exploiting women's unpaid work in the same way as community care policies that advocate a 'mixed economy' of welfare (Finch, 1984). In some accounts, the community development focus on 'meeting needs' serves to incorporate and neutralise resistance to state policies whilst at the same time protecting the interests of welfare professionals (Armstrong, 1982). It is important not to see women's health activism simply as a resource for health policy. The strength of women's health groups is often in their autonomy and in the fact that they provide an alternative, sometimes critical, perspective on women's health issues.

TOWARDS A FEMINIST HEALTH PROMOTION?

Health promotion, whether individually or collectively focused, may be an appropriate strategy for enhancing women's health. However, inappropriate health promotion activities may have negative effects, by misconstruing or ignoring women's health needs, or by provision which is inaccessible or which reproduces health damaging tendencies. The promotion of women's health is a complex issue that demands a range of responses. However, it is important that strategies address women's needs rather than construct women as carers. Gender stereotypes that view caring and nurture as 'natural' to women only serve to legitimate policies that create unhealthy pressures at the same time as failing to provide resources for caring.

Gender inequalities affect all women, although of course women's experience of sexism differs significantly. Women are also divided by other dimensions of inequality structured by class, ethnicity, sexuality and disability. Both the common characteristics that constrain women's lives and the divisions between them need to be recognised in health promotion. The current vogue for addressing women as consumers able to exercise personal choice over lifestyles and health care services is inappropriate, given the constraints on most women's lives.

Collective approaches to health promotion are often favoured by commentators who are critical of individualistic strategies. However, sexist assumptions may also influence collective policies which are not necessarily underpinned by a social model of health. Social policies that aim to promote health may have the effect of penalising the most vulnerable, as the example of poor women smokers and increased tobacco taxation demonstrates. The health risks that women face often arise from the wider environment which is structured by gender as well as other inequalities. Stronger Government controls on tobacco promoters, which would reduce smoking rates without penalising smokers, are therefore increasingly advocated by a very broad spectrum of interested parties.

Collective negotiated strategies are relatively untested, and have many features that may appeal to feminist practice. Even in today's economic climate, there are opportunities for community development approaches which have the potential to provide more appropriate and sensitive services for women. However, it is important that such approaches do not exploit women as unpaid and invisible carers for the community.

Feminist health promotion may embrace diverse strategies, and the women's health movement has demonstrated the importance of diversity and a multiplicity of practice. However, integration is needed in order to avoid generating contradictory pressures on women. There is a need to consistently challenge the assumption of responsibility without power that characterises women's relationship to health promotion in order to transform this relationship into one which offers positive health through support for real choices.

ACKNOWLEDGEMENTS

We would like to thank Lesley Doyal, Alison Gilchrist and Kate Wood-house for their useful comments on an earlier draft of this chapter.

Chapter 6

Developing anti-racist health promotion strategies

Jenny Douglas

INTRODUCTION

The aim of this chapter is to outline, review and provide a critique of health promotion approaches and perspectives that have been developed and adopted to promote health with black and minority ethnic communities in the UK. A review of changing historical perspectives in relation to social policy and black and minority ethnic communities will be attempted and strategies proposed for developing anti-racist practice.

Health promotion approaches cannot be divorced from dominant prevailing ideologies and social policies in relation to 'race' and the presence of black and minority ethnic communities in the UK. The last forty years have seen the development of social policies relating to black and minority ethnic communities that have adopted a range of perspectives or models: assimilation, integration and multiculturalism. The chapter proposes an anti-racist approach to health promotion. Although anti-racist approaches have emerged and developed from within black and minority ethnic communities, these have never been fully sanctioned by Government health policies and strategies. The chapter also explores the possible reasons for this.

MODELS OF SOCIAL POLICY

Assimilation, integration, multiculturalism

Britain has always been a multiracial or multicultural society; however, it is only relatively recently that the terms 'multiracial' and 'multicultural' have been used. Although there have been black people living in Britain since at least the sixteenth century, the usage of these terms coincides with the growth in Britain's black population during the postwar period. Early references in the medical literature in relation to the health concerns of black communities in Britain focused on 'Port Medicine', with a concentration on exotic diseases and the importation of illness (Johnson,

1984). Within the model of assimilation prevalent during the early 1960s, black and minority ethnic people were perceived as 'dark strangers' with exotic cultures and diseases. The emphasis in relation to health education approaches during this period was to provide information to black and minority ethnic communities on aspects of lifestyles and cultures that were seen to be deviant to dominant white cultures. Hence there was a proliferation of literature on family planning, the diets of Asian communities and tuberculosis. The underlying assumption was that the cultures of black and minority ethnic groups were deviant and hence lifestyles and cultures should change so that black communities could be 'assimilated into' dominant white cultures.

During the mid- to late 1960s a model of social integration emerged whereby it was envisaged that black communities would not completely abandon their cultural heritage and a philosophy of 'tolerance' and recognition of cultural differences was seen to underlie prevailing social policies. Alongside this the reports relating to the health of black and minority ethnic communities started to increase with an emphasis on physical and cultural differences. An increased number of articles appeared on sickle cell anaemia trait, thalassaemia and other haemoglobinopathies. The response in relation to health education and health promotion was an increasing literature on cultures and lifestyles of black and minority ethnic communities. The use of 'culture' and cultural explanations in relation to health experiences and health care arrangements increasingly became the focus in a social policy movement away from integration and towards multiculturalism.

'Culturalist' perspectives attempted to explain the health status, health experiences and health behaviour of black and minority ethnic communities in the UK purely in terms of culture, often comparing black and minority ethnic cultures to white majority cultures in a detrimental way such that the beliefs and values of minority cultures were undervalued. This is clearly demonstrated when reviewing research examining the health status of black and minority ethnic communities in the 1970s and 1980s when health problems were often attributed to the behaviour of individuals or their culture, rather than their socio-economic position (Donovan, 1984). The focus of attention was on illness and diseases affecting black and minority ethnic communities and much of the research was underpinned by a bio-medical model (Douglas, 1992). The main health concerns reported and researched were tuberculosis, rickets, mental illness, perinatal mortality and low birth weight syndrome. These topics reflected areas perceived as problems by (predominantly white) health professionals and researchers and were not necessarily areas of concern to black and minority ethnic communities themselves. Having defined these areas as problematic, health professionals and researchers then attempted to attribute these health concerns to aspects of lifestyles, family patterns and organisation and the culture of black and minority ethnic communities.

The models of health education developed were based upon educative approaches – the assumption that by providing black and minority ethnic communities with information, lifestyle and behaviour would change. Deficit models of health education and some early health education programmes and strategies were not sensitive to cultural beliefs and practices and in some instances were in opposition to the cultural beliefs and practices of some black and minority ethnic communities. Such approaches 'blamed the victim' or their culture for poor health, and did not address social and economic factors contributing to the poor health status of many black and minority ethnic communities.

A major health education campaign developed in the late 1970s and early 1980s was the Rickets Campaign, which was launched by the Department of Health and Social Security in 1981. This was the first health education campaign to be targeted at black and minority ethnic communities and was identified as an issue for action by medical researchers and health professionals and not by the communities themselves. The increased incidence of rickets in some Asian communities during the 1970s was attributed to poor diets and lack of knowledge about vitamin D, foods or restrictive cultural practices that prevented women and children from exposing their skin to sunlight. The health education campaign focused upon giving Asian communities advice on how to change their traditional diets to British diets, which were thought to be higher in vitamin D content. Critiques of the Rickets Campaign (Sheiham and Quick, 1982) outlined the significant difference in Government policy in relation to rickets in Asians – where health education strategies were employed to change behaviour of Asian communities – and in white populations in Britain during the Second World War, where the problem was addressed by fortification of particular foods like margarine with vitamin D. This clearly demonstrated that while in Asian communities rickets was perceived to be a problem associated with cultural preferences and practices, in relation to white populations rickets was perceived to be a problem associated with poverty. An examination of this particular issue is useful in that it highlights difficulties with the use of cultural explanations. There is, for instance, an inherent assumption that Asian communities are homogeneous, and that all Asian people have had the same cultural, religious, historical, social, economic and political influences. This approach ignores the existence of wide variations in religion, class and gender.

The emphasis on culture, in relation to developing health and social policies, meant that black communities were often perceived as being problematic rather than the inflexible, ethnocentric health services. Pearson (1986) contends that black people and minority ethnic communities have always had a second-class image in the health services, first as migrant workers and second as patients having different diets, languages, lifestyles and religions.

Following an integrationist perspective, the developing emphasis on acknowledging cultural differences in terms of the health care needs of black and minority ethnic groups in Britain brought with it initial difficulties associated with the development and perpetuation of stereotypical descriptions and assumptions about black and minority ethnic communities and cultures (Henley, 1979; 1980; Henley and Clayton, 1982). The 1980s saw a burgeoning literature attempting to define, describe and explain black and minority ethnic cultures and practices. It was also during the late 1970s and early 1980s that black communities started to campaign about the need for specific health education information. Sickle cell anaemia and the campaign for appropriate services is one such example.

It could be argued that the cry for action around inherited blood disorders presented a further reinforcing of approaches to health and health education in relation to black communities based upon the medical model, thus directing attention from wider health concerns affecting large sections of black communities by focusing attention on a specific disorder affecting only a small section of such communities. It also provides an example of the lack of response to a clearly defined need and the institutionalised racism of the NHS (Prashar *et al.*, 1985).

During the 1980s several authors posed critiques of cultural perspectives arguing that they could not adequately explain the health experiences of black communities in Britain. Although culture will affect health behaviour, health experience and experiences of health services, an explanation based solely upon culture excludes the importance of socio-economic, political and material factors upon health and health experience (Thorogood, 1990). Many studies seeking to examine the experiences of black communities in relation to health have excluded socio-economic categorisation and have used broad generalisations based upon stereotypes of cultural difference and bio-medical models of 'race' and ethnicity. Further, culturalist perspectives have often represented black and minority cultures as being deviant or alien and have ignored the dimension of gender.

Another drawback of the multicultural approach was the emphasis on developing health promotion programmes and resources targeting particular minority ethnic communities to the exclusion of others. Whilst there were many resources and materials developed for some Asian communities, there was relatively little information or resources available for Chinese, Vietnamese (Mares *et al.*, 1985) and African-Caribbean communities (Douglas, 1987; 1992). This demonstrates the difficulty of starting from the point of examining cultural difference rather than building upon a common experience of racism and discrimination.

Materialist perspectives

A more adequate framework for understanding the health experiences and health status of black and minority ethnic communities is to incorporate the dimensions of class and socio-economic position. Several studies have demonstrated that black people occupy a disadvantaged position in British society (Brown, 1984). As is well known poverty has been demonstrated to have detrimental effects upon health (Townsend *et al.*, 1988), and therefore the health of black people in Britain will be determined to a large extent by their socio-economic position and experience of racism and racial discrimination in all aspects of their lives (Donovan, 1984; Pearson, 1989).

In the next section I will briefly review current approaches to health promotion for black and minority ethnic communities against the back-cloth of the WHO's *Strategy of Health for All by the Year 2000* (WHO, 1981) and the Department of Health's White Paper *The Health of the Nation* (Department of Health, 1992a). I will examine the present multi-cultural approach and outline its shortcomings. I will conclude by proposing a strategy for developing anti-racist practice in health promotion.

THE CURRENT CONTEXT

Most present health promotion programmes and strategies for black and minority ethnic communities emanate from a multicultural perspective. The campaigns are based upon the notion that black and minority ethnic communities have different cultures and languages and that these should be recognised and valued. Although the stress on cultural and linguistic difficulties with regard to the health services obscures more fundamental issues in relation to equality of opportunity to good health, some authors argue that these approaches have paved the way for health workers to develop more effective channels of communication with black and minority ethnic communities (Tunon, 1986; Rocheron, 1988). A number of policy documents on the health needs of black and minority ethnic communities produced in the late 1980s highlighted the need for culturally sensitive approaches.

A failure of the multicultural approach is the lack of acknowledgement of the material causes of ill health in black and minority ethnic communities in relation to poverty, discrimination, poor housing, poor working conditions, employment and racial harassment. All of these areas have been documented (Brown, 1984) but have had little impact upon the development of health promotion programmes that address issues relating to inequality. It is almost as though by addressing the health promotion needs of black communities from a cultural perspective issues of inequality were also being dealt with.

The WHO strategy *Health for All* strives to reduce and eliminate inequalities in health. Although many health authorities purport to follow this strategy, it has never been endorsed by the British Government in any real way (Ahmad, 1993b). It is significant to note that nowhere in the literature accompanying and supporting the WHO's strategy is any reference made to black and minority ethnic communities and migrant communities in Europe. Thus although equity underlies the approach of *Health for All*, there is no recognition of this in relation to racial discrimination and racism. The publication of *The Health of the Nation* (Department of Health, 1992a) did not acknowledge inequalities in health in relation to poverty, class, culture or gender and returned to a medical model approach with a focus on five key areas.

DEVELOPING ANTI-RACIST HEALTH PROMOTION STRATEGIES

In this section I will examine and make recommendations about anti-racist health promotion strategies. Anti-racist perspectives acknowledge that inequalities in health emanate from structural factors that affect the lives of black communities which in turn impact upon health and health experience. Developing anti-racist health promoting programmes must be done within a context of a wider strategy for equal opportunities.

Many health authorities purport to involve local communities in decision making and determining key priorities and to have policies based upon community development principles. An examination of these approaches demonstrates that local communities are rarely involved in decision making processes and, where it has been developed, black communities are rarely consulted and more rarely actively participate; 'local voices' are rarely 'black voices'. Health promotion is based upon the principle of community participation and development and hence mechanisms to actively involve black and minority ethnic communities should be developed. A review of health promotion programmes for black and minority ethnic communities demonstrates that where health authorities and other organisations reported programmes based upon principles of community development, in reality they were health promotion programmes based upon traditional methods that were simply delivered in community settings. Thus, such programmes had not involved black and minority ethnic communities, groups or individuals in their conceptualisation, development or implementation. Black communities should be involved in developing health promotion programmes and in setting the agenda in relation to priorities for action. This means that assessment of

health needs should involve black communities in determining methodologies and research programmes for health needs assessment.

Many health promotion programmes and projects targeting black and
minority ethnic communities are funded on a short-term basis and often
seek to employ black officers. Such health promotion officers are often
employed at a level where either they do not have access to decision
making processes or are excluded from them. This again marginalises
health promotion activities for black communities, and often issues
addressed in mainstream health promotion programmes such as poverty,
women's health, coronary heart disease programmes and so on are not
reflected in the specific health promotion programmes developed for
black and minority ethnic communities. The knowledge and experience
that black/minority ethnic health promotion officers have are not widely
acknowledged and officers may find future promotion difficult.

Nationally, there has been no clearly defined strategy for promoting
health for black and minority ethnic communities from the Health Education Authority (HEA) or Health Education Council (HEC) before it.
The response of this organisation to health promotion and black communities is worthy of a detailed research project and a chapter in itself.
More recently the HEA has attempted to undertake research studies on
the lifestyles and health behaviour of black and minority ethnic communities as many lifestyle research projects have not included black and minority ethnic communities (Blaxter, 1990). A recent Department of Health
guide, *Ethnicity and Health* (Balarajan and Raleigh, 1993), documents
epidemiological information on patterns of illness in black and minority
ethnic communities in relation to the key areas identified in *The Health
of the Nation*. However, no reference is made to the material conditions of
black and minority ethnic communities and the role that socio-economic
circumstances may play in the differential patterns of illness.

CONCLUSIONS

An anti-racist perspective, while recognising differences and diversity that
exist within black and minority ethnic communities within the UK, seeks
to place racism and material disadvantage as the central common experience of black communities. Health promotion programmes and activities
adopting this approach must be developed by black and minority ethnic
communities. This means black communities must be involved actively in
their development and implementation. As the many factors that impinge
upon health are not under the direct control of health services, local
networks across a range of voluntary, statuary, community and business
organisations must be developed. The evaluation of health promotion
programmes by local black people must be encouraged; too often health
promotion programmes are never effectively evaluated and rarely by

people who are supposed to benefit from the programmes (White and Bhopal, 1993). Health promotion programmes must be developed within a wider organisational framework that has equality and equity as core values. This said, it must also be recognised that health promotion in itself cannot overturn the injustices in society as a whole that contribute to the racism and discrimination that affects the health of black and minority ethnic communities. Health promotion can only be part of a much wider movement towards a just and fair society.

Chapter 7

The modern and the postmodern in health promotion

Michael P. Kelly and Bruce Charlton

INTRODUCTION

This chapter is organised around distinctions between the modern and the postmodern, modernisation and postmodernisation. It is argued that health promotion contains within its theory and practice contradictory elements both of modernism and postmodernism. Out of these contradictions arise a range of inconsistencies and tensions. We suggest that these tensions can themselves be analysed as the products of the time and context within which health promotion, as a distinctive set of public health practices, emerged. Resolution of this tension is suggested with reference to the sociological problematic of the interaction between agency and structure. We begin with a sketch of the modern–postmodern distinction.

MODERNISM AND POSTMODERNISM

The modern world and modernism were initially distinguished from the traditional or ancient worlds by social theorists. The traditional world was stable and controlled by religion and magic. The modern world in contrast was progressive and was dominated by rationality and science. The progress and advance of the modern was legitimated by a belief in the ultimate discovery of scientific truth. *Post*modernism refers to a range of movements and ideas at the core of which is a critique of modernism's underlying assumption that knowledge and science might in some sense be unified methodologically and epistemologically and that an ultimate bedrock of truth, fact or morality might be discovered (Seidman and Wagner, 1992). One of the central ideas of postmodernism, therefore, is an abandonment of the notion of science travelling towards an end in which it will eventually have a complete correspondence with reality (Rorty, 1982).

Modernity is the habitat of normal science (Kuhn, 1970) and of rationality applied to physical or social problems (Lyotard, 1984). Postmodernity is the world of aesthetics, the deconstruction of conventional social arrangements and of experimentation in culture, art and life (Lyotard, 1984; Bauman, 1992a; Featherstone, 1988). In postmodern thinking, present social and moral arrangements mark a fundamental break with the past. Life is viewed as chaotic and its understanding as contingent. Instead of progress there is just change. Reality is defined as paradoxical, ambiguous, uncertain and open-ended (Featherstone, 1988). The philosophy of *difference* is central to postmodernism (Lemert, 1992: 24–5). This contends that the distinctions between truth and falsehood, essence and appearance, the rational and the irrational must be dissolved because there is no ultimate guarantee or reason for these differences outside and prior to language (Snyder, 1988: xii-xiii).

HEALTH PROMOTION, POSTMODERNISM AND VESTIGES OF MODERNISM

Postmodernism as described here has a tremendous resonance with health promotion both in theory and in practice (Kelly *et al.*, 1993a). The rejection of medical science as the basis of health promotion and reliance instead upon notions of holism and complete social and physical wellbeing is premised upon a social model of health. The philosophy of *difference* finds echoes in themes of empowerment and the politicisation of health issues (WHO, 1986a). The rejection of ultimate truth is represented in the highly relativistic notions of health that pervade health promotion with its emphasis on aesthetics and subjectivity. The deconstruction of scientific knowledge is to be found in various so-called community-driven identifications of health issues and the reconceptualisation of disease, not as the malfunction of organs and organisms but as the ideological expression of medical power and dominance and an account of the powerlessness of particular segments of the population.

A range of keynote statements about health promotion makes this abundantly clear. The original definition of health in the World Health Organisation constitution (WHO, 1946) described health as a complete state of physical, mental and social wellbeing. This definition set the original postmodern motif because it dissolved the Kantian distinction between science, art and morality. Health was to be seen as a fusion of the true, the beautiful and the good with subjective fulfilment. Taken to its logical conclusion this definition marks the break with medical science. It may be argued that health promotion is premised upon a *social* concept of health, and not a medical or mechanistic microbiological view of health and illness. This is an explicit rejection of the scientific paradigm and an attempt to introduce other types of analysis. The Lalonde Report (1974), which is often taken as a seminal text in the origins of the health promotion movement (Hancock, 1993; Tsouros and Draper, 1993), suggested that the major determinants of health were considerably greater than the sum of medical and hospital care and scientific and bureaucratic knowledge. The Lalonde Report proposed the idea of health fields as determinants of health. The health fields were environment, lifestyle and biology (Hancock, 1990: 2). Matters of medicine and of science thus became extended into matters of political and social science and of politics and values. Although Lalonde is more an extension of the medical model than a transformation, it none the less weakened it and has been used to justify attacks on it.

The next key statement is the Alma Ata Declaration of 1977 (WHO, 1978). This argued: first, that governments have a responsibility for the health of their people; second, that it is the right and duty of people individually and collectively to participate in the development of their health; third, that it is the duty of governments and health professionals to provide the public with relevant information on health matters so that they can assume a greater responsibility for their own health; and fourth, that there should be individual, community and national self-determination and self-reliance in health matters (Catford, 1983). The implication was clearly that health is primarily about politics, not in the traditional sense of class or ethnic power struggles, but as an issue-based matter. Moreover, a clear separation of science and politics is heralded as a necessary precondition for progress. This is in stark contrast to the modernist way of doing things in which science and politics are conjoined.

The next major landmark in health promotion is usually taken to be the *Ottawa Charter for Health Promotion* (WHO, 1986a). This defined health promotion as 'the process of enabling people to increase control over and improve their health'. This, so the argument went, involved a recognition that power and control are the central issues in health promotion. The critical task was to become the empowerment of communities to define an agenda for themselves in health terms and to seize the political initiative so to do (McKnight 1985; Rappaport, 1977). The *Charter* went on to argue that the process was premised upon certain prerequisites for health, namely peace, shelter, education, food, income, a stable ecosystem, sustainable resources, social justice and equity. The *Charter* also outlined five overlapping and interactive means of making health promotion happen: building healthy public policy, creating supportive environments, strengthening community action, developing personal skills and reorienting health services. Political action would lead to a strong foundation for health. This social and political programme has formed the major plank in the overall objectives of health promotion since that time.

In 1988 a major meeting in Adelaide produced a consensus statement that described healthy public policy as characterised by an explicit concern for health and equity in all areas of policy and by an accountability for health impact. It was acknowledged that using public policy to achieve equity in health would involve diverse government departments including agriculture, education, social welfare, housing and economics. Creating support for this wide involvement in health required, it was said, an innovative and effective system of political accountability that would make visible the positive and negative effects on health of sectors other than health services.

We suggest, following Stevenson and Burke (1991), that health promotion may therefore be viewed in part as a discourse of the new politics with its implicit and explicit critique of the attempts to improve society by a marriage of science and the bureaucratic state. Its discourse of enhanced power for civil society *vis-à-vis* the state, for decentring and democratisation and its reordering of social priorities are part of the same package. The attacks on medicine, the appeals to empowerment and the emphasis on communities defining their own health needs, all resonate to a postmodern tune.

However, within this postmodern discourse there also lurk vestiges of modernism. Despite claims to the contrary, the approaches to health promotion used by the WHO in particular, and by the many national and local health promotion agencies in general, remain locked into technicist, scientific and, above all, expert-driven practice. The key statements above proclaim the principles of health promotion in the name of the community and indeed espouse principles of community involvement in the process of health promotion (for example WHO, 1988a). However, they retain a practice pushing in the exactly opposite direction (Kelly, 1989). The documents *Research Policies for Health For All* and *Priority Research for Health For All* (WHO, 1988a; 1988b) for example, emphasise the idea of community involvement in setting the research agenda. However, one searches in vain to find evidence of community involvement in the WHO's deliberations on the matter and in the production of these texts (Kelly, 1989; 1990). Experts still appear to be in control. The reliance on such expertise is modernism and normal science writ large. In the face of a problem, the solution proposed here is finding the right kind of expert with the appropriate kind of knowledge to solve the problem. It is not decentred and it is not based on a philosophy of difference. Communities remain marginalised and invisible – other than in the rhetoric.

CRITIQUE

Perhaps it is hard to imagine that the health promotion agenda could be anything other than expert-driven. The leap to decentring and abandoning normal science in favour of bringing in lay people to define problems and suggest methodologies for their solution is just too great, too difficult and too uncomfortable (Davies and Kelly, 1993). Indeed, it is paradoxical even for experts to discuss how to abandon expertise! Our argument is with the humbug that makes claims for a social model of health and then uses this as a stick with which to beat medicine in order to claim the moral high ground. Our contention is that science (including social science) remains at the heart of public health and health promotion. For all the talk of empowerment, the experts remain firmly in control of the discourse of health promotion.

Our second observation is that the much-vaunted break with the medical model is more apparent than real. Antonovsky (1985; 1987) has argued that there is a dominant assumption which runs through most scientific endeavours whether practised by physicists or physicians. This is the assumption of system. When a physicist analyses an atom or a molecule, or when a physician examines a human body, they use systems and structures to make sense of what they see. Systems are used very profitably as heuristic devices. They are also particularly helpful in understanding when pathologies occur. Seeking out the cause of system disintegration is central to the scientific endeavour. Of course, advanced scientific thinking does not reify systems and an appreciation of the failure of systems, and the problems of observing systems are central features of scientific knowledge. Social science is also based on systems-type thinking. By this we do not mean that all of social science is dominated by some variant of structural-functionalism or Marxism. Rather, we mean that nearly all major social science paradigms (be they concerned with markets, institutions, group dynamics, the unconscious, or power) contain within them notions of the systemic. Social scientists focus on system breakdown in the same way that natural scientists do. Their concerns are with imperfect markets, dysfunctions in organisations, social pathology in groups, development of neurosis and exploitation in relationships, for example. What is essentially similar between the natural and social sciences is, according to Antonovsky, a doctrine of cause in which bad precursors have bad outcomes. The social model of health is, in this regard, no different to the medical model. In the medical model the pathogens are microbes, viruses or malfunctioning cellular reproduction. In the social model they are poor housing, poverty, unemployment and powerlessness. The discourse may be different but the epistemology is the same. The social model is not, in our view, an alternative to a discredited medical model. It is a partner in crime and a very close modernist relative.

In an effort to emphasise the social model of health in health promotion, some rather damaging things, sociologically speaking, have been done in its name. We suggested above that the scientific version of systems thinking and the important heuristic power of systemic ideas were tempered with a realisation that systems are changeable, that their existence is at least in part a function of their manner of observation and that system chaos is part of the scientific lexicon. In other words, systems have a status not as real things in themselves but as a means to a scientific end. The error in a good deal of health promotion, as exemplified by the key statements reviewed above, is that the social system is reified. It is described as acting on people in a highly deterministic fashion. Unemployment *causes* ill health. Deprivation *causes* disease. Society (the biggest system of all) is held to be at fault. The system is found to be working in a way that disadvantages particular groups. The individual is relegated to being nothing more than a system outcome, not a thinking and acting human. The person is the victim of a system.

Not only is such thinking based upon a crude and vulgarised version of sociology, it is also premised upon an ecological fallacy. There are, of course, significant statistical associations between poverty and ill-health and unemployment and disease. But to argue that everyone who is poor or unemployed will inevitably become ill would be to apply to individuals characteristics of the aggregate group (the ecological fallacy) and to attribute a causal relationship between qualitatively dissimilar entitles – namely social structure and biological function. Interestingly, much public health medicine is based on the same kind of principle. The preventive medicine strategy of making mass interventions to reduce the population rate of coronary heart disease, while having negligible effects at the individual level, uses the same causal argument as society causes disease, only in reverse! It is a pleasing irony that the proponents of the argument that society causes disease should end up in precisely the same epistemological position as those public health epidemiologists whom they frequently affect to despise.

We suggest that mixing the modern and postmodern in health promotion has produced a politics and ideology of health, that veers incoherently between the scientific and the chiliastic. In this potent cocktail, muddle is compounded by muddle. The confusion begins with the concept of positive health. The idea of positive health as the goal of health promotion is seductive. It is held to be more than the reciprocal of disease. It is supposed to represent a fulfilled and fully functioning quality of life, lived to the full and to be enjoyed by all in a state of complete social, physical and mental wellbeing. Health is transformed from being a neutral idea relating to non-pathological physical functioning, and the fulfilment of ordinary social roles, into a social and political value, loaded with moral connotations. To be healthy is a good thing, not because it means the absence of pain and suffering, but because it is a fundamental good. Health is thus reformulated as a basic human right (Crawford, 1977: 668). Health in this sense has expanded out of control. Cut loose from disease-based definitions of science and medicine, it has become a commodity and like all commodities is available in the marketplace (Charlton, 1993a: 34–5). If individuals and communities do not have it, then this must be someone's fault, and depending on your favoured political position that 'someone' is either government or society (health as a right) or an imperfect market (health as a commodity). As a moral position, as a normative principle and as a political statement, health thus becomes a very convenient way of attacking one's political opponents. Health is defined as a great liberating force. It is linked to power and domination or to socio-economic arrangements.

Intriguingly, much of the rhetoric about health in this sense carries a freight of modern and scientific assumptions, that somehow through technical, political and economic means, it is inevitably possible to achieve health and if health is not achieved this must be due to some sin of omission. This therefore links together several great enlightenment concerns. The belief is that the application of knowledge, linked to political will, will essentially result in progress. Health thus brings together progress, improvement, science, economics and politics in a mixture of righteousness (Crawford, 1977: 668).

But the transmutation of what was a biological idea based on the notion of equilibrium to a political value must not go unchallenged. Health, and the concern of governments for the health of their populations, is not a cultural universal. There have been many historical epochs when rulers felt no responsibility for the health and wellbeing of their people (Charlton, 1993b). This was not just because they did not possess the means to do anything about health even if they had wanted to, it was simply that there was no moral imperative on them to do so. Certainly with the arrival of potentially effective public health interventions a technology to do something became available. But the existence of the technology, the means, or the partial means, does not create the moral imperative. What health promotion assumes is that the desire for health *is* a moral imperative. Yet it is no more so than any other human right or commodity. Rights and commodities are actually context specific and culture bounded.

Our next objection is to the idea of some kind of Utopian world in which everyone can be healthy. Much of the critique of health differentials, for instance, starts from an assumption that the state of health is natural, and any departure from health requires explanation (Charlton, 1994). This flies in the face of every piece of knowledge and information that biological, medical and social science has accumulated in the last two hundred years. Being alive is intrinsically risky. The human body is a delicate and vulnerable organism which is subject to a multitude of noxious assaults from the moment of conception. Humans have to survive this risky world (Charlton, 1994). These risks are microbiological, genetic, environmental, social and physical. The world is a thoroughly dangerous place. Over the last few hundred years the world has been made a relatively safer place and human organisms can be protected, up to a point, from many communicable diseases, from each other and from environmental hazards. Social and political systems have developed which, in certain parts of the globe, facilitate a safer civic society too. But all of this is partial. New communicable diseases emerge, standard immunisation programmes can never guarantee immunity and may themselves carry risks. Even the most developed societies have social problems and physical violence lurks not far beneath the surface of the most civilised of Western democracies. At the same time as health has improved, humans have been devising the most mind-boggling forms of mass destruction, and industrialisation has levied a heavy toll in hazards, pollutions and environmental damage. War remains commonplace and famine is endemic throughout much of the world.

There is not, and there can never be, a risk-free environment, an idea which is widely understood by the lay public (Frankel *et al.*, 1991). The role of microbes is a case in point. Many are lethal to humans, yet a bacteria-free world would be a dead world. And there is no freedom from the ultimate fate of dying. To be human is to engage in behaviours to which dangers are routinely attached and to be exposed to environments which carry risks or have negative effects on the organism. What is of course entirely feasible are attempts to reduce risks, to limit potential damage and to produce a relatively *healthier* population. It is quite possible to develop policies, to implement them and to evaluate their health benefits scientifically (Young, 1993). But a *healthier* population is not a healthy population in any absolute sense. It is a pity that so much health promotion seems to promise absolutes and is not tempered by more careful relativism.

There is one final objection to the overarching philosophy of health promotion. The emphasis on health is at the expense of an emphasis on disease, and more particularly an emphasis on pain and suffering. To place the emphasis on achieving a better world some time in the future is to downplay the here and now, and is to underemphasise the real problems that real people have (Kelly, 1990). In our view, this is the true moral high ground. Time, energy and resources should be directed into an alleviation of actual pain and suffering as a priority rather than into creating imaginary political systems in the future. This is a political statement by us of course, but we suggest that existing medical technology and social engineering can achieve a great deal, and certainly a great deal more than idealised political visions. This is so if we think of the value of clean water and working sanitation on the lives of infants in developing countries where diarrhoeal illnesses have a high prevalence. It is true when we appraise the effect of warm, dry housing on the health of populations in the public sector housing schemes in Great Britain. It is true if we think of the profoundly beneficial effects of drugs like the H_2 blockers on diseases of the upper gastro-intestinal tract, and of the effects of antibiotics on a whole range of illnesses. These are things that can be done immediately. They are much more effective than inventing Utopias and than attacking governments, doctors and social planners for failing to provide them.

SOME THEORETICAL CONSIDERATIONS

Given these inherent problems, why and how has health promotion emerged as such a compelling idea? Sociologically speaking we suggest that health promotion with all its tensions and confusions is a product of a social epoch which is best described as a period of *postmodernisation.*

In a recent book, Crook and his collaborators (Crook *et al.*, 1992) provide a useful analysis of the distinctions between modernisation and postmodernisation. Sociology, they argue, has been characterised since its inception as the study of, and theorising about, processes of modernisation. Indeed sociology is itself a product of modernity. Comte, the inventor of the word sociology, saw progress and the dominance of science as inextricably linked. In the works of the classical sociological writers – Durkheim, Weber and Marx – the elements in modernisation are signalled and they remain, according to Crook *et al.*, the means of understanding the process. These are: differentiation, rationalisation and commodification.

Differentiation is most closely associated with Durkheim. His interests in the division of labour and the ways in which simple forms of social organisations (mechanical solidarity) are transformed into complex forms of social relationship (organic solidarity) are explored with reference to the social bondings of groups and individuals, the form of legal organizations and the nature of norms and values (Durkheim, 1933). These themes are further explored in his study of suicide (Durkheim, 1952) in which the links between the individual and particular forms of social organisations are demonstrated. In *The Elementary Forms of the Religious Life*, (Durkheim, 1915), Durkheim examines the relationships between knowledge, social structures and belief. The underlying motif through each of these works is a focus upon the *forms* of social organisation and its mode of differentiation.

In Weber's historical and organisational sociology he focuses on rationalisation (Weber, 1930; 1947; 1948; 1961). This he finds in forms of commercial and productive relationships, in religious practices and in organisational forms of power and authority. For Weber, rationalisation was a paramount historical process manifested in an array of real historical events, *and* an idealistic process because rationalisation accompanies a disenchantment with the world meaning the loss of spontaneity, charisma, joy and passion.

In Marx's encyclopaedic writings, arguably the most enduring contribution is not his emphasis on class conflict, nor the economic theory he used to explain conflict and social development. It was rather his understanding of the commodification of life and the closely related ideological structure that sought, or functioned, to conceal that commodification (Marx, 1962; Marx and Engels, 1970). Marx observed the reduction of everything to a cash nexus. This encompassed not just formal economic or commercial transactions, but the nature of social life itself. The relationships between classes, men and women, and nation states are all ultimately reducible to a commodity value, itself determined by the nature of the productive and reproductive process. Meanwhile such commodification is clouded from view by ideologies masquerading as science, art, culture and history which prevent these commodified relationships being revealed for what they are.

For Crook and his colleagues (Crook *et al.*, 1992) differentiation, rationalisation and commodification are the backbone of modernity. Crook and colleagues then take us a step further and demonstrate that the forms of social organisation of contemporary Western society are an elaboration and an exaggeration of differentiation, rationalisation and commodification. This elaboration and exaggeration *is* postmodernisation. The contemporary world is *hyper*-differentiated, *hyper*-rationalised and *hyper*-commodified. We have not suffered a fundamental break with the past, as postmodernist theory claims. On the contrary we are working out trends which have their roots deep in early modernity.

The *hyper* processes are to be found in varying degrees in a range of spheres of culture, state formations, gender and class inequalities, politics, work and production and science. In culture, form and content give way to pastiche and admixture, the state's power is delegitimated in various ways (such as privatisation and deinvolvement), gender and class inequalities blur, politics become issue-focused, work and production is detached from the industrial process and science is distrusted and undermined (Crook *et al.*, 1992: 36–41).

With respect to health promotion, various elements of these characteristics of postmodernisation are easy to discern. In the world of postmodernisation the function of the state as a tool of social and economic regulation shrinks and state power diminishes. In health promotion the emphasis is, in some versions, on sub-state formations such as communities, cities, localities and/or an emphasis on individual responsibility (rather than state responsibility) in others. The appeal of supra-state formations such as the WHO to issue-based politics in the explicit way the Ottawa Charter is framed, for instance, is evidence of similar processes at work. Health promotion is an excellent example of the new politics of postmodernisation. Health is *the* issue; health has, as we suggested above, an appeal far beyond governments or national politics. It thus becomes a convenient tool for attacking and delegitimating state functions – national and local.

Hyper-differentiation is represented in terms of the plurality of competing paradigms and practices in health promotion, which are drawn from public health, sociology, education and psychology (Bunton and MacDonald, 1992) and the proliferations of various occupational groups who view health as *their* territory – doctors, nurses, health educators, environmental campaigners, community development workers, occupational health specialists and so on.

Hyper-rationalisation is represented by the ever-increasing tendency to push health into the private sphere. Whereas once upon a time someone visited a doctor only if they felt ill, the health promoter colonises the private world of even the well person, invades their private life and their sexual, dietary, drinking and tobacco habits, the way they bring up their children, the type of transport they should use to go to work; and provides a rationale for such invasions on the grounds that everything is potentially a health issue! The health promotion philosophy *in extremis* is much more intrusive in people's lives than ever medicine was. It will even attempt to empower communities when the community had never thought of it for themselves.

Hyper-commodification is represented by the idea that health is a consumer good. Health is fashionable; it is linked to beauty, to appearance, body image, to fitness. In the modern period health became a right. In postmodernisation health became a consumer good to be bought and sold like everything else. In the British National Health Service this is now fully institutionalised as health promotion became part of the internal market (Yen, this volume): a service to be purchased! Health is about lifestyle and lifestyle is about consumption (Bunton and Burrows, this volume; O'Brien, this volume).

We suggest therefore that health promotion emerges when it does, in the form that it does, as part of the process of postmodernisation. Its frenetic activity, and its tensions and contradictions are postmodernisation in action.

CONCLUSIONS

The most powerful critiques of health promotion have come from diametrically opposed political viewpoints. On the one hand, the radical right has castigated health promotion on a variety of grounds which have included its anti-libertarianism, its nanny-state mentality, its interference with the operation of free market forces, its social engineering, its locatedness in middle-class liberalism and so on. Writers such as Skrabanek (1991; 1992), various right-wing think-tanks (Social Affairs Unit, 1991), and a range of like-minded critics have found fault with the principles of health for all, health promotion and so on.

On the other hand an equally penetrating critique has originated in the work of left-wing writers who have pointed out that all the wishful thinking about behaviour transformation and Utopian systems misses the most fundamental point of all about the distribution of illness in society (Davison *et al.*, 1991). This is the presence of a steep social class gradient and its origins in inequalities in power, wealth and status. The problem is formulated by left-wing writers as a structural one, in which worrying about personal dietary habits, alcohol consumption, safer sex and the rest is regarded as displacement from the main issue, which is that health and disease are products of social differentials and the real effort should go into tackling the disease, not the symptoms.

We have sympathy with both views and enjoy the apparent paradox that leftward and rightward thinkers should be so united in their scepticism (Davison and Davey Smith, this volume). This is in fact no paradox. If we trace both free-market libertarianism and Marxist-oriented attacks on the social structure back to their roots, they are of course the same. Both are derived from the philosophy of utilitarianism and the classical economics of the late eighteenth and early nineteenth centuries. Utilitarian thinking with its underlying philosophy of freedom (of markets, or individuals) stands in marked contrast to the authoritarianism and ideological flights of fancy of health promotion.

The central problem, as we see it, is that the health promotion movement has become a political movement, without resolving the key philosophical problems at the heart of both rightward and leftward thinking, namely the reconciliation of free will *and* determinism in explaining human behaviour. For health promotion, free will is held up as a guiding principle, embedded in notions of empowerment and facilitation, while at the same time defining the social structure as acting *on* people in a deterministic way. This becomes especially tortuous when describing the behaviour of oppressed groups. Here the emphasis is on social determinism among the oppressed while maintaining a place for the idea of free will among non-oppressed groups (such as health promoters). Empirically this may be the way the world seems to operate, and politically it may make considerable sense to construct things in this way. But theoretically and epistemologically it does not work. Either we are all free or are all socially determined. You can't have it both ways. Because the health promotion movement wants it both ways, it finds itself attacked both by the free will school of the right and the structuralists of the left.

However, help is at hand. In modern social theory some very important attempts have been made to acknowledge the interaction between free will and determinism, or, put into the contemporary sociological discourse, between agency and structure. The work of Giddens (1982) is most illuminating in this regard. In his idea of structuration the two faces of structure and agency are brought together as a way of providing a thoroughgoing account of human behaviour. The theory may be summarised as follows. Humans exist in a physical and social world which is structured in various ways. These structures set the limits as to what may be achievable at any given moment or in a lifespace for any particular individual. The social structures are not, however, physical in any sense. They only exist through the discourse in which they are expressed, maintained and reproduced. Those structures of language and discourse provide a stock of knowledge which allows humans to operate within them. They provide for a grammar or a vocabulary of taken-for-granted meanings and assumptions that constrain human actions and behaviours. But those constraints are not externally imposed; they are internally imposed in so far as the social actor guides his or her own action within the parameters established in their understanding of the social world. By participating in social discourse, humans contribute (albeit usually in a small way) to the transformation of that discourse. Humans are therefore both the makers of their own destinies and are constrained by the destinies so created. Both human action and social structure are thus fixed into the analysis in terms of the meanings which are produced and reproduced in those self-same structures.

Health promotion might reflect upon Giddens' theoretical work, and seek to develop means of reconciling and understanding human behaviour in the light of his contribution to sociology. Human agency (choice, imagination and ingenuity) is necessary for understanding and predicting human action, but it is not sufficient. Sufficient understanding would include a consideration of social structure, the individual's comprehension of this structure, and how it impinged upon their life. Such a dynamic and reciprocal analysis of the individual set into *context* ought to be at the heart of health promotion (Kelly *et al.*, 1993b). Developing this, and making it work, is the task ahead.

Health promotion in its present form is riven with contradictions in theory and in practice. This state of affairs is exacerbated by the moralising zeal characteristic of the field which serves only to impair reflection. The result has been a failure to confront critique. This strategy has not worked – the critics will not go away, and they are winning the debate. Without acknowledgement of its own contradictions, and serious efforts to resolve them, health promotion deserves no better than to remain the object of critiques by both left and right. As things stand, out-argued, outflanked and outnumbered, it is doubtful how long health promotion can last as a viable discourse and practice.

Chapter 8

The baby and the bath water

Examining socio-cultural and free-market critiques of health promotion

Charlie Davison and George Davey Smith

SOME SHARED THEMES IN CRITIQUES OF HEALTH PROMOTION

The last fifteen to twenty years have witnessed major developments in preventive medicine. These developments have been characterised by an increasing acceptance in medical and political circles that the common chronic diseases of middle and later life constitute the principal health issues of industrial societies (Lalonde, 1974). Attendant on this realisation came the idea that the maintenance of health and the avoidance of illness (rather than attempts to cure it) should move to the centre stage of health policies, with the concomitant shift in focus of medical activity from the sick to the well. While the practice of preventive medicine is plainly not 'new' in any sense, a particular style of 'healthy living' advice has tended to move to the forefront of state health policy (see, for example, DHSS (1976a), HEC (1983), Department of Health (1992a)). It is this relatively recent wave of health education and health promotion activities, and the various critiques that have developed with them, that are the focus of this chapter.

One of the striking aspects of this movement is that the conceptual landscape of prevention has become characterised by the emergence of a clear policy agenda based on the management of mass behaviour change. This policy agenda has been built on foundations laid down by a variety of fitness, nutrition and hygiene movements which characterised nineteenth and twentieth century urban life. A major difference in the modern versions, however, is a new scientific respectability derived from the postwar development of population epidemiology and the 'discovery' of a range of behavioural causes of hitherto quite mysterious forms of death such as heart attack and cancer. This process involved the replacement of prewar concepts regarding broad social determinants of health status and health potential, acting from early life through the life course, with an individualised and largely asocial notion that the behaviours of adults were all important (Kuh and Davey Smith, 1993). While the very disease constructs on which this transformation was predicated can be seen as historically specific, or even politically necessary (Bartley, 1985), the implications of aetiological theories restricted to adult behaviour for apportioning responsibility for disease causation and disease avoidance are more transparently functional.

These developments have brought to the fore the concept of 'lifestyle' – a loose aggregation of behaviours and conditions encompassing body size, body shape, diet, exercise and the use of drugs both legal and illegal. Improving the 'lifestyle' of the population, indeed, soon became the major goal of the movement. The implementation of the mass behavioural change deemed necessary by these developments was first entrusted to a somewhat amorphous professional grouping initially known as 'health education' and, later, 'health promotion'.

Almost from the outset, the movement to change the 'lifestyle' of the population attracted severe criticism from some quarters. The suggestion that the cardiovascular diseases and cancers which account for a high proportion of deaths in industrial societies are due to the 'lifestyle' of sufferers automatically brings forth the issue of culpability. If a disease is preventable by adopting (or desisting from) certain behaviours, then it follows that victims of such disorders are at least partially to blame for their predicament (Crawford, 1977; Radical Statistics Health Group, 1987).

The moral discomfort attendant on blaming the sick becomes more acute if the scientific basis of the identification of 'lifestyle' as pathogenic is questioned. A recurring theme in critiques of behavioural preventive medicine has, therefore, entailed the questioning of the processes that attribute a specific proportion of disease to 'lifestyle' causes (see, for example, Sterling (1978) and Davey Smith and Shipley (1991)).

The core idea of such critiques has been that health education and health promotion have, by overemphasising the individual's role, been guilty of oversimplifying disease causation. While this type of criticism is normally associated with a political standpoint to the 'left of centre', such oversimplification is plainly infuriating to some who espouse a more right-wing individualist position. Le Fanu, for example, writing on the promulgation by health educators of the concept of a 'healthy diet', observes that:

> In all their self-righteous admonitions to the public, they appear blind to the serious consequences of their propaganda – that it misinforms the public about the complexity of disease, trivialises tragedy and blames patients for their illnesses.
>
> (Le Fanu, 1986: 124)

Other critiques have been more specific, holding that the elements of multi-factorial aetiologies that involve personal 'lifestyle' have been given too great a weight and the elements involving forces and conditions that are outside or greater than the individual (heredity, environmental contamination, poverty, etc.) have been officially 'played down'. From a political perspective well to the left of Le Fanu, the multicausal orthodoxy of modern social and preventive medicine has been identified as being subtly ideological. Multicausal theories allow for many factors – social, psychological, physiological, behavioural, etc. – to interact in the production of disease. Such an approach appears to give space and weight to psycho-social influences and thus escapes victim blaming in a simple sense. This balance is, however, more apparent than real, since interventions go on to target what is seen as most tractable, which is generally individual behaviour. Furthermore, responsibility can be shifted by a motivated reweighting of different factors. As Tesh points out, in a trenchant critique of multifactorial theories:

> This equal weighting of causes also means that those who have something to lose from prevention programmes can insist that the factor for which they have no responsibility is the real cause. For example, asbestos companies can insist that smoking is the real cause of lung disease, and cigarette companies can insist that occupational exposure is the culprit. Smokers can take their pick. The multicausal web by itself offers no clear challenge to these positions.
>
> (Tesh, 1988:24)

For Tesh only the recognition that the apparently value-free multifactorial aetiological theories are nothing of the kind can produce effective health promotion. Preventive medicine, according to this type of critique, must be predicated on the notion that social structure determines exposure, which determines outcome.

Likewise, our own research into the relationship between epidemiological findings, public perceptions of risk and health promotion messages in the field of heart disease prevention led us to the conclusion that

> health education has never come to terms with the complex relationship between the individual and the collective in the field of health and illness. Rather it has opted for a form of worthy dishonesty based on . . . half-truth, simplification and distortion.
>
> (Davison *et al.*, 1991: 16–17)

Oversimplification is one of a pair of common strands in critiques of behaviour-based prevention. The other is the recognition that the priorities of health education are often at odds with the ways in which the general public thinks, feels and acts in relation to health. This 'clash of cultures' theme involves more than one way in which health education and health promotion are out of step with the wider society.

In the first place, the pursuit of good physical health may simply not be at the top of personal agendas:

Lifestyle interventions and social engineering are disruptive to people's lives and raise the political question – do people want to be healthy? This is not a facetious question, as there is always a price to be paid for health. For some people health is not a top priority. Some actively seek high risk pastimes such as rock climbing, fast driving or excessive drinking. Alternatively, health may be accorded a relatively low priority by individuals suffering psychological difficulties or social deprivation. In such circumstances we must ask whether people have a right not to experience interference, and whether health promoters are in danger of becoming a 'safety police'?

(Kelly and Charlton, 1992: 223)

The suggestion here is that good health does not have a unique value, rather that it exists in a conceptual field that allows it to be, from time to time, compared with and even exchanged for other desirable goals. This balancing or 'trading' to maintain life quality is to be found in many recent research-based accounts of how 'lifestyles' are constructed in everyday life (see, for example, Graham (1987), Mullen (1992), Backett (1992) and Backett *et al.* (1994)). The clash between the idea of 'trading off' health chances for life quality on the one hand, and a 'medically recommended' lifestyle on the other, is colourfully described by Charlton:

Such is the crusading zeal of these 'safety nazis' that they do not require firm, well-validated evidence before making their sweeping recommendations (or laws) about how we should live or spend our money. Just the suspicion of danger is enough to precipitate action, 'just to be on the safe side'. There is an explicit denial of the citizen's responsibility for their own health. The Health Police's model for human goals and behaviour is as restricted as its own views: they refuse to believe that rational and free citizens will choose to smoke tobacco, drink alcohol, eat 'too much' of the 'wrong' foods and refuse to go jogging, even though they know these things may be bad for their health. Normal people, as a matter of course, will happily sacrifice the possibility of an illness in the long term against present enjoyment.

(Charlton, 1993a: 32)

Differences between the priorities and cultural values belonging to preventive medicine on the one hand, and popular culture on the other, are illustrative of a more pervasive discourse involving the perception and management of risk. In the field of toxic waste hazards, for example, Brown (1992) reports that local and professional perceptions were essentially dissimilar, and that 'the public' attached quite different meanings and values to their assessments of possible or probable health damage. A more clearly political analysis, in which the clash between local and imposed priorities is seen as 'a form of resistance' is provided by Balshem

(1991), in her investigation of how an American working-class community reacted to a lifestyle-based anti-cancer campaign. In similar vein, our own research into heart attacks suggests that a public culture of prediction and explanation is often more salient than 'official guidelines' when lifestyle behaviours are planned or assessed (Davison *et al.*, 1991).

Gifford points out that the overall tension between professional and lay assessments of probable harm are due to the fact that medical calculation involves the mapping of information collected from aggregated populations on to the unique trajectory of a single life (Gifford, 1986). The desire to guide the behaviour of the individual by referring to the average experience of the group has been crucial to the development of a predictive concept of 'risk' (Hacking, 1990). Risk, and its management, has, in turn, become a *leitmotif* of the mission to control future events that has characterised social life in the 'late modern' period (Giddens, 1991). Nelkin and Tancredi suggest that these conceptual developments have led to a situation in which the thinking of medical and other élites has become dominated by an

> actuarial mind set [which] is designed to limit liability and requires calculating the cost of future contingencies, taking into account expected losses, and selecting good risks while excluding bad ones. The individual must therefore be understood actuarially, that is with reference to a statistical aggregate.
>
> (Nelkin and Tancredi, 1989: 9)

DIFFERENT CRITICAL PERSPECTIVES

It is our aim in the second section of this chapter to examine the differences between the philosophical bases and policy outlooks of a variety of critical perspectives. We illustrate this field by constructing a 'spectrum' of perspectives, which ranges from collectivist analyses of social life on the one hand to individualist positions on the other. In Tables 8.1 and 8.2, comparisons are made of the ways in which different types of critique articulate their positions in relation to two basic public health issues and two specific 'defining moments' in public health policy that occurred in 1993.

We have illustrated the spectrum by choosing to describe four points on its length. On the collectivist end, we have labelled a 'Fabian or Marxist' perspective. This type of approach is best represented by the positions taken up by groups within the political left and organised labour, in conjunction with sympathisers amongst academics and professionals (see, for example, Radical Statistics Health Group (1987) and Tesh (1988)). The key notion for this tendency is that the distribution of health and illness is a direct function of the social, economic and political relations that define society. The key fact is that the health of those in professional and managerial occupations is generally good, while that of manual and service workers is generally poor. This position, therefore, concentrates on highlighting the health-damaging effects of poverty, work, working conditions and the environmental degradation of working-class living spaces. There is often little dialogue with professional health education or promotion, so few basic premises being shared that communication would be difficult, even if it were sought (which it generally is not).

Our next illustrative position is one we have labelled 'new public health'. A representative statement of this perspective could be found, for example, in the *Ottawa Charter for Health Promotion* (WHO, 1986a). Here, some of the underpinning ideas of the social democratic tradition are recognised, in particular the notion that health and health experience cannot be understood in isolation from economic and social conditions. The new public health position, however, identifies environment and lifestyle as key mediators in the relationship between structural position and health experience and classifies both as potential areas for interventions. The crucial area of operation for promotional activities is the place where environment and culture create lifestyle, hence there is much interest in such conceptual areas as 'stress' on the one hand, and such concrete issues as damp housing on the other.

The position we have labelled 'health of the nation' takes its name from the UK Government paper of the same name (Department of Health, 1992a). In terms of preventive medicine policy and outlook, there are two main features of this tendency. First, the importance of individual responsibility has been underlined by the integration of individual behaviour change and the surveillance of health-related behaviour into the formal workload (and payment structure) of general practitioners (Department of Health and the Welsh Office, 1989). Second, the social and economic contexts of lifestyle and behaviour in disease causation have been implicitly downgraded by the setting of blanket national targets for behavioural change (Department of Health, 1992a).

The fourth position, at the individualist extreme of the spectrum, is labelled 'free market'. A good example of this is the analysis of smoking choices in the light of Bayesian decision theory provided by Viscusi (1992). The key issue here is that the individual freedom of citizens to make personal choices and so design their own lifestyles is the type of inalienable right established by the political and constitutional movements that grew out of the enlightenment. The state, in whatever guise, therefore, has no right to intervene. A similar philosophical perspective is to be found underpinning the various papers concerning food and health promotion published by the Social Affairs Unit, a right of centre 'think tank' of some importance in UK policy circles in the 1980s (Anderson,

1986). The political component of the free market position is illustrated by the memorable words of one professional pro-smoking campaigner (the Director of the pro-tobacco group FOREST quoted in Davey Smith (1993)) who dismissed health promotion as an attempt by 'the social-working class to dictate the lifestyle of the real working class'.

Table 8.1 Approaches to two 'basics' of public health

Collectivist ⟶ Individualist			
'Fabian' or Marxist' perspective	'New public health' perspective	'Health of the nation' perspective	'Free-market' perspective
Production of disease The distribution of illness is a function of the relationship between the economic and social spheres of collective action	Many diseases are linked to personal behaviours and shared environments. These exist in a social/ political context	Many of the major diseases of industrial society are rooted in personal behaviours which have a social and geographical distribution	If illness is caused by personal behaviour, then individuals are free to choose health or illness from a range of lifestyle options
The design of health promotion interventions Interventions should aim at social justice and material improvement – equity in health will follow	Sensitive attention to pathogenic lifestyles – 'empowerment' of individuals and communities to choose health	Pathogenic lifestyles to be tackled at source – i.e. the individuals who do them should be identified and persuaded to change	The idea of 'an intervention' involves the notion of collective conformity. Health can only be chosen by individuals, not by a 'nanny' state on their behalf

Before referring to Table 8.2, some words of explanation are required. Harry was an English man whose case dominated the mass media and was hotly debated throughout the UK for a short period in 1993. Harry's predicament was that he was diagnosed as needing a heart bypass oper-ation, but was excluded from the waiting list on the grounds that his continued smoking would make surgical intervention unlikely to succeed. The story came to symbolise a wider question – that of whether partici-pation in 'risky lifestyles' constitutes grounds for differential access to

Table 8.2 Reactions to two 'defining moments' of 1993

	Collectivist ───► Individualist			
	'Fabian' or Marxist' perspective	*'New public health' perspective*	*'Health of the nation' perspective*	*'Free-market' perspective*
Reactions to Harry	Harry should receive his rightful treatment. His heart trouble has as much to do with his social disadvantage as it does his smoking	Harry's smoking is not his problem alone. He should get treatment. But this is a useful debate as it helps to stigmatise smoking and so facilitate behavioural change	Give up smoking or lose your right to treatment. The exclusion of the self-inflicted sick could save valuable NHS resources for more deserving cases	The moral and political issues should be shelved. Both smoking and medical treatment should be treated as a consumer's freely made 'product choices'
Reactions to Reg	A cynical ploy to make profit from misery. Ban it	Tobacco advertising must be banned. Smoking must be stigmatised. (Plus a grudging admiration of some very clever advertising)	Opposed to any encouragement of smoking. But we must stand by commercial freedoms. Tobacco companies should be socially responsible	Individual citizens can and must decide for themselves. Companies can advertise freely, so can health campaigners if they want to. It's a free country

health care. It brought the issue of self-infliction to the centre stage of political and public discussions of health and the prevention of illness.

Reg was a figure in a poster cigarette advertisement. He was 'an unattractive, ageing, bald man ... making a stupid face, eyes half closed, lips pressed together in an idiot's leer' (Leith, 1992). Reg, through his various poster appearances, made pithy and humorous comments on topics of public interest, such as party politics ('if you drop ash on the carpet you won't be invited again') and the greenhouse effect ('my tomatoes do better under glass'). He clasped a cigarette in his fingers and epitomised most successfully the image of a smoker as someone who has enough common sense and *joie de vivre* to be able to hear health warnings but make his own decision to enjoy life to the full. After inciting strong opinions and reactions on all sides, Reg was eventually withdrawn on the grounds that research had shown that he was particularly appealing to young people and thus in contravention of the tobacco industry's voluntary guidelines on cigarette advertising (Hastings *et al.*, 1994).

CONCLUSION

In this brief examination of the various political and philosophical bases that underpin critiques of health education and health promotion, we have suggested that some key points are shared across a broad spectrum from individualist to collectivist positions. These shared themes include criticism for the misrepresentation or distortion of epidemiological findings, the tendency to blame victims and sufferers for their illnesses and the unproductive and conflictual relationship with non-medical or 'lay' culture.

Beyond these shared points, however, we have attempted to show how serious differences exist between different critical perspectives, not only in terms of the philosophies that underpin critiques of health education and health promotion, but also on specific policy issues. While individualist tendencies suggest that the entire project of health promotion is neither possible nor desirable in a free society, collectivist approaches are based on the opposite point of view. In the individualist perspective the entire enterprise of health promotion is flawed and the only acceptable policy would be one based on the free availability of epidemiological risk information and total liberty of product choices. From the collectivist point of view, the individualisation of responsibility and the attempts at cultural engineering have been wrong-headed, but these flaws do not destroy the overall prevention project.

At heart, the differences lie in the fact that collectivist positions display an overriding concern with equity in life chance and exposure to the risk of illness. Health promotion, from this point of view, represents a potential weapon in the battle against socio-economic inequalities in health. Individualist perspectives, on the other hand, eschew any such societal approach to health and discount health promotion as unwarranted state intervention in the life of the citizenry.

Our suggestion is that, in spite of a coincidence of interest and a concordance of views in some areas, it is important that those who seek to modify and improve health promotion do not agree too strongly with those who seek to destroy it. We conclude with the recommendation that the valuable babies of social justice and an even distribution of health chances are not thrown out with the dirty bath water of authoritarianism, victim blaming and the cruel illusion of individual control over illness and death.

Part III

Knowledge, risk and health promotion

Chapter 9

The case of passive smoking

The case of passive smoking

Peter Jackson

INTRODUCTION

The concept of passive smoking, the involuntary inhalation of other people's tobacco smoke, has transformed the boundaries within which tobacco smoking can be discussed (Chapman *et al.*, 1990). No longer the sole concern of the smoking self, the public consumption of tobacco is now projected as an activity with serious implications for the health of others. For example, the Health Education Authority (HEA) estimates the risk of lung cancer from passive smoking to be '50 to 100 times greater than the risk of lung cancer from exposure to asbestos' (HEA, 1991a: 3). More directly, the Government's Independent Scientific Committee on Smoking and Health (ISCSH) quantifies a 10–30 per cent increased risk of lung cancer in non-smokers exposed to environmental tobacco smoke (ISCSH, 1988), an assessment further conceptualised in terms of 600 lung cancer cases per year in the UK (King's Fund, 1988).

That these specialised, scientifically based calculations influence everyday knowledge and experience needs little elaboration. Increasingly cast in terms of intrusion and constraint rather than as a legitimate means of expression, smoking is now restricted in many of the public spaces of social life: on public transport, in shops and banks, theatres, cinemas and restaurants. Airline passengers, for example, can now travel on 'fresh air' services and diners can consult a list of establishments guaranteeing not only a non-smoking environment but also a fine for those guests who fail to observe it (*Today*, 29 May 1991). The workplace too has been 'sanitised'. Reflecting and reinforcing a wider trend, the UK division of the Ford Motor Company adopted a no-smoking policy in its offices from January 1990 (Gabb, 1990). Indeed, most office staff who smoke can no longer do so at their desks and a local government worker was recently compensated for the apparent long-term effects of exposure to the cigarettes of those who once did (*The Independent*, 28 January 1993). The conceptual boundaries of tobacco smoking, then, are being redrawn, our ways of thinking and acting transformed in relation to a fundamental shift in the scientific understanding of smoking and its effect upon the health of non-smokers.

However, whilst we are prompted by these developments to think differently about the effects and consequences of tobacco (ASH, 1993), we are not encouraged to think differently about the ways in which the new scientific facts underpinning them are produced:

> There's mounting scientific evidence that passive smokers face not just a social nuisance but an actual threat to health.
>
> (BSS, 1991: 3)

> Until the late 1970s, scientists thought that passive smoking was no more than a social nuisance to most non-smokers. But research now shows that it's more than just a nuisance. It can also be a health hazard.
>
> (HEA, 1987)

Thus, research 'now shows' and evidence 'mounts' as science progressively reveals and accumulates knowledge about a preexisting reality. Moreover, in relation to a logic and method of enquiry traditionally seen to be based upon the 'norms' of universality, communality, disinterestedness and scepticism (Merton, 1973), that knowledge is distanced both from the interests and actions of those who identify and promote it and the wider social context in which those practices are pursued and accomplished. The conclusions of science 'are true and necessary', as Galileo put it, 'and the judgement of man has nothing to do with them' (Galileo Galilei, quoted in Mulkay (1979: 20)).

This chapter explores the emergence and development of those conclusions fundamental to the construction of passive smoking as a threat to public health. Challenging the assumptions of scientific realism, it locates the production and content of this new medical knowledge in discourse and process. In so doing, however, a number of commitments have been made which require clarification.

First, the Mertonian idea that the content of science is an inappropriate subject for sociological investigation is obviously challenged. The 'judgement of man' (sic) has everything to do with the conclusions of science – a judgement in itself which helped underpin the shift in sociology from the 'weak programme' to the 'strong programme', from the sociology of science to the sociology of scientific knowledge (Mulkay, 1979; Stehr and Meja, 1984). In general terms, this approach perceives the procedures and conclusions of science as cultural products and argues that empirically based scientific facts are not simply determined by the physical world but also depend upon socially derived assumptions (Mulkay, 1984: 79).

Second, it is recognised that this perspective frames a considerable range of ontological, epistemological and methodological commitments.

Bartley (1990), for example, distinguishes the 'laboratory studies' (Latour and Woolgar, 1979; Gilbert and Mulkay, 1984), which examine the micro-processes and discursive tensions underpinning the emergence, nego-tiation and establishment of scientific facts, from the wider 'social interest' model of explanation (Barnes and Shapin, 1979). Here, 'forms of know-ledge or knowledge claims are to be expected to evolve with changing *interests*, as the material position of the social groups changes' (Bartley, 1990: 376; emphasis in the original). Finally, offering a wider, processual account of the development of scientific knowledge, there is the work of Thomas Kuhn (1970) and Ludwig Fleck (Fleck, 1979; Cohen and Schnelle, 1986), to which one might add the very different conclusions of Norbert Elias (1971; 1978).

This chapter is particularly influenced by the theoretical ideas of one of the latter group of writers: Ludwig Fleck's constructionist account of the genesis and development of scientific facts. According to Fleck, scien-tific knowledge is produced not by accessing and accumulating facts about an external reality but in relation to a set of theoretical interpretations of that reality. He calls these theoretical frameworks 'thought styles'. Thought styles contain the rules for thinking, rules of possibility that facilitate the formation of certain ideas and render others unintelligible. Moreover, thought styles are seen as 'collective phenomena' (Cohen and Schnelle 1986: xi), made manifest by 'thought collectives', groups of people sharing a particular way of thinking. Thus, scientific knowledge is collective knowledge, inseparable from the wider assumptions, traditions and relations of time and space. And, as a consequence, it follows that if collective scientific thought is socially patterned, by social institutions and historical processes, so changes to that knowledge must also be patterned (Lowy, 1988). Thus, for Fleck, as White explains, 'there is no linear progression of knowledge, only a changing in thought styles' (White, 1991: 61); a gradual process in which new sets of questions are provoked and new forms of scientific understanding developed.

Informed by these ideas, this discussion examines some of the mechan-isms involved in the development of one particular aspect of that under-standing: the construction and legitimation of passive smoking as a scientifically 'proven' threat to public health.[1]

ACTIVE SMOKING AND MEDICAL KNOWLEDGE

The phenomenon of passive smoking is a relatively new concept in medi-cine, a new way of thinking about tobacco and its capacity to impact upon health. Medical perceptions of the consequences of active smoking however, are more firmly established. This section briefly discusses the genesis and development of some of those ideas, ideas which confined the health effects of smoking to the individual smoker (WHO, 1971: 5) and rendered the concept of passive smoking unthinkable. The chapter then moves on to address the question of how a once unthinkable idea, that of passive smoking, is now not only possible but prominent.

In 1920 the annual number of lung cancer deaths in England and Wales was estimated at 250. By 1960 that had risen to over 10,000 (Taylor, 1985). During the latter part of that period tobacco smoking was identified by medical science as the most significant contributory factor in the transformation of these mortality patterns and trends (Doll and Hill, 1950; Royal College of Physicians, 1962). Today this assessment appears natural and inevitable – 'the rise in lung cancer accompanied the rise in cigarette smoking' (Taylor, 1985: 3) – the incontestable outcome of a rational logic of enquiry. However, as Fleck reminds us: 'Cognition is neither passive contemplation nor the acquisition of the only possible insight into something given. It is an active relationship . . . an act of creation' (Fleck, 1986a: 49).

Moreover, as we noted earlier, it is a 'collective act', culturally conditioned by a given 'thought style' (Fleck, 1979). Thus, when Doll and Hill and their contemporaries (see Taylor (1985)) identified and sought to explain the increasing prevalence of lung cancer, the way they thought as medical scientists reflected and reinforced the way they saw the world around them. And what they 'saw' were new patterns of disease mapped out on the discrete bodies of the population. The locus of health over which medicine presided was changing, the individual body it seemed was more susceptible to lung cancer in the 1950s and 1960s than it was in 1920. The norm was shifting. As Scheper-Hughes and Lock instruct us, however, the concept of *the* body, let alone that of a normal body, is 'both naturally and culturally produced, and . . . anchored in a particular historical moment' (Scheper-Hughes and Lock, 1987: 7). Its classification as 'matter' and subsequent separation from mind or spirit, for example, owes more to Cartesian philosophy than to nature and yet this opposition is incorporated by Western culture as a fundamental natural 'fact' of human life. Indeed, it is one that informs and underpins a whole host of oppositions embedded in our epistemology: nature and culture, reason and passion, individual and society, even the real and the unreal (Scheper-Hughes and Lock, 1987: 8–11). As Fleck puts it: 'we look with our own eyes but we see with the eyes of the collective' (Fleck, 1986b: 137).

To return, then, to the scientific collectives of the 1950s, to the increasing incidences of lung cancer in the bodies of the population and the questions asked by medicine in an attempt to understand the phenomenon. Those questions, as we have seen, were motivated by changing trends in the statistical representation of the medical subject, the discrete, physical body. More 'subjects' were breaking away from the medical norm, thereby challenging the bedrock of the medical knowledge base. Traditionally, medicine is seen to respond to such challenges by expanding that base, pushing back the boundaries of its knowledge through discovery and revelation. If we accept, however, in the spirit of Fleck's constructivist sociology, that the questions asked in a piece of research 'largely determine the type of data gathered' (Boissevain, 1974: 215), and that those questions are in themselves stylistically shaped and informed, then data gathered must also be data produced. Intimately associated with the socio-cultural context framing its development, all knowledge expresses the forces that make it intelligible. It is 'stylised'. Socially contingent and historically conditioned, observation and theory are bound together in a web of interdependencies. Consequently, the way in which we think not only determines the way in which a problem is perceived, but also the boundaries within which it can be resolved. And for the investigators of the 1950s and 1960s those boundaries reflected and reproduced a particular conception of the bio-medical scientific model.

For example, in their 1950 study Doll and Hill classify their participants as 'cases of carcinoma of the lung, stomach, or large bowel' (1950: 741). This has a number of implications. First, they represent the individual body, in a diseased state, as the self-evident concern of medicine, the natural subject of medical investigation (Hahn and Kleinman, 1983). As we have seen, this reduces the patient to an aggregate of mechanisms and systems, an asocial individual body. Second, the diseases to which this body is subjected are themselves seen to possess a natural existence, an existence beyond that of the categories and perceptions of medicine. This provokes and naturalises a particular perception of the causation of the diseased state. Doll and Hill, for example, seek explanation in terms of an external causative agent impacting upon individual health: 'The great increase in the number of deaths attributed to cancer of the lung in the last 25 years justifies the search for a cause in the environment' (Doll and Hill, 1950: 747).

Such ideas are more than 'passive contemplation'. They are 'stylistic' productions, made intelligible in relation to a particular contextual logic and rationality: a way of knowing that constructs a space between social actors and their 'environment', thereby encouraging the detachment of patients from their social contexts. A way of knowing that further reduces patients to their bodies and 'objectively' defines health in terms of the absence of professionally defined disease in those bodies. And, thus, a way of knowing that produces knowledge not by accessing an independent reality but in relation to stylistic interpretations of that reality.

To summarise so far: it has been argued that the epidemiological detection of disease patterns in the 1950s and 1960s, and the subsequent discovery of tobacco smoking as a significant influence upon them, were themselves patterned by the scientific stylisations of health, disease and the body. Data were not simply gathered; they were produced in relation to a particular way of seeing and knowing the world. Medicine's thought style represents the world and produces its facts in relation to those representations. However, the very stylistic frameworks that enabled medicine to see and represent the health hazards of tobacco smoking so clearly also rendered other possibilities invisible; 'the increasing ability to perceive necessarily involves a mounting loss' (Cohen and Schnelle, 1986: xxi). Thus, whilst medical science could 'see' the consequences of tobacco smoking for the individual body, it was less able to theorise connections between those bodies. The following section explores the genesis and development of those new scientific ideas that encouraged medicine to make those connections, to ask new types of questions and, thus, to produce new forms of knowledge about the relationship between tobacco and ill health.

PASSIVE SMOKING – EARLY THOUGHTS

Although tobacco has been a prominent subject of medical investigation since the 1950s, references to passive smoking are relatively few in the medical literature prior to the early 1970s. Some research was conducted around this time; Speer studied the relationship between cigarette smoke and the 'subjective symptoms' of eye irritation and headaches (Speer, 1968) and Colley et al. (1974) looked at its impact on the incidence of pneumonia and bronchitis in children during the first five years of life. Others assessed possible relationships between ambient smoke and allergies (US Department of Health, Education and Welfare, 1979) and the tolerance of exercise in angina patients (Aronow, 1978). However, the literature lacks coordination at this point and apart from aesthetic considerations, which have been articulated since King James's famous Counterblaste To Tobacco ('a custome lothsome to the eye, hateful to the Nose', quoted in Gabb (1990: 14)), the medicalisation of passive smoking was minimal.

By 1988, however, a review of the 'health hazards of passive smoking' (Eriksen et al., 1988) produced over 80 references, many of which made the link with disease. How was this shift in perception made possible? Dosimetry has been identified as the first step.

> Without some idea of the relative amounts of smoke constituents to which passive smokers and smokers are exposed, it is impossible to judge accurately evidence of the alleged health effects of passive smoking.
>
> (Lee, 1984: 190)

However, without some idea that things can be reduced to their constituent parts in the first place, there can be no notion of dosimetry. Passive smoking may be a new conceptual development but it is based upon an established way of thinking. As we have seen, medical discourse reduces and disaggregates; it fragments before it rebuilds and produces its facts. And this logic is apparent here as medical science strives to articulate the possibility of tobacco smoking as a threat to public health. For Lee such strivings are in vain – 'there is no convincing epidemiological evidence that exposure to environmental tobacco smoke (ETS) results in an increased risk of lung cancer, heart disease or any other disease in non-smokers' (Lee, 1992: xix) – but the point that is principally of interest here is the conceptual transformation of tobacco smoke taking place in relation to the dosimetric argument. Smoke itself is being subjected to the scientific gaze, but in becoming a focus of scientific attention it is 'recreated' by it, reproduced in style. Thus, no longer just smoke, it is now represented as an aggregate of 'smoke constituents', a representation that is projected as inevitable and given. For example, Shephard argues that: 'it is usual to distinguish the discontinuous or particulate phase of cigarette smoke from the continuous or gaseous phase' (Shephard, 1982: 17). The particulate phase includes such substances as tar, nicotine and benzene and the gaseous phase consists, amongst others, of carbon monoxide, ammonia and hydrogen cyanide (ASH, 1989). Such classifications, of course, are not inevitable. They are only 'usual' within the frameworks of scientific medical thought but, as with the notion of the discrete, mechanistic body and the independent existence of disease, these productions are projected as natural and incontestable. More importantly, they also redefine the possibilities of understanding.

For example, having deconstructed tobacco smoke and projected this new knowledge as 'usual', beyond reproach, the Surgeon General then reassembles the parts to fabricate a new type of whole. She or he conceptualises the constituents of cigarette smoke in terms of three different categories: most likely health hazards (for example, tar), probable health hazards (for example, nitric oxide) and possible health hazards (for example, benzene) (Shephard, 1982: 18–19). A number of points are worth noting here. First, this new way of perceiving tobacco smoke reinforces the notion of scientific enquiry as a linear process of revelation and knowledge accumulation. Medical science may not yet know the full extent of the ill-effects of inhaling nitric oxide but it does 'know' that it is probably more hazardous than inhaling benzene. Mapped on to this hierarchy of hazards, then, are images of the progressional nature of scientific understanding, its capacity to gradually reveal and accumulate facts about external phenomena. Second, the reconceptualisation of substances such as nitric oxide as 'probable health hazards' popularises esoteric knowledge. Thus, scientific facts are packaged for popular consumption and so too, of course, is the logic of enquiry that produced them.

However, despite these developments, dosimetry is largely considered to have been ineffective as a mechanism for conceptualising and communicating the idea that tobacco smoke was harmful to the health of non-smokers. Lee (1984), for example, challenges the methodology of several studies designed to measure levels of exposure to environmental smoke (for example Repace and Lowrey, 1980). And Horsfield, discussing the issues involved in general terms, points to the complex relationship between such variables as exposure to the numbers of people smoking and cigarettes smoked and concludes that 'there is no satisfactory way of measuring passive smoking' (Horsfield, 1984: 179). However, this 'stylistic' concern, whilst promoting certain ideas also prevents others from being articulated. Crudely, a way of thinking that constructed knowledge in relation to discrete bodies in a state of disease was ill-equipped to theorise connections between bodies, particularly those *out* of disease. Problems of measurement, therefore, were accompanied by the more pressing sociological problem of the *invisibility* of the passive smoker. The subject of enquiry, necessarily one characterised by connections and relations, appeared difficult to conceptualise in a discourse that reduced and disaggregated the phenomena of its investigations. Dosimetry reflected and reinforced those constraints.

Following Fleck, however, we have seen that scientific knowledge is socially produced in relation to the possibilities of style rather than by accessing an external reality. Scientific facts are creations, productions of a particular way of seeing. Such productions, however, are more than static creations. They also feed back into the processes of construction and impact upon those processes. Thus, the stylistic processes that initially facilitated the connection between cigarette smoke and disease and further led to the reconstruction of that smoke in terms of its chemical components, were themselves influenced by the nature of their productions. Further, one of the most significant productions underpinning medicine's shifting perception of the relationship between tobacco smoking and ill health is the idea that a cigarette generates two types of smoke.

MAINSTREAM AND SIDESTREAM SMOKE

Roughly 75% of the smoke from a lit cigarette goes straight into the air as sidestream smoke. The smoker inhales 25% as mainstream smoke, and breathes half of this out again. In total, 85–90% of cigarette smoke gets into the air which others breathe.

(GASP, 1982:1)

The categories of mainstream and sidestream smoke are by no means the only ones produced by medical discourse. Shephard, for example, identifies four other types of smoke generated in the act of smoking a cigarette; smoulder-stream, glow-stream, effusion-stream and diffusion-stream

(Shephard, 1982: 24). These constitute subcategories of sidestream smoke, further classifying it in terms of its point of departure from the cigarette (filter, burning tip, etc.) and in relation to different stages of the smoking process. However, the sidestream/mainstream dichotomy, conceptually differentiating all unfiltered smoke from that drawn through a cigarette prior to inhalation, is considered to be the most significant scientifically.

Sidestream smoke, it is argued, is chemically distinct from that of the mainstream. It has a higher carbon monoxide content and is comprised of smaller particles which 'are more likely to deposit in the most distant alveolar portions of the lung' (Byrd *et al.*, 1989: 209). Thus, sidestream smoke is projected as a natural entity, something 'out there', like disease, beyond the categories of medicine. Following Fleck, however, we can see that, far from simply being 'out there', sidestream smoke is also very much a product from within, a concept related to the processes and perceptions of stylised scientific investigation. Science reduces and reconstructs the phenomena of its investigations and produces rather than reveals its facts. And with the distinction between mainstream and sidestream smoke what is produced, in a sense, is smoke for the smoker and smoke for the non-smoker – 'the smoker inhales mainstream smoke . . . [the rest] gets into the air which others breathe' (GASP, 1982: 1). Two types of smoke; two types of social actor. Now we're all affected, both by tobacco smoke and the categories of medical science.

The implications of this new scientific 'fact' for the promotion of passive smoking as a threat to public health are significant. The early attempts to construct environmental tobacco smoke as a threat to public health foundered, principally, because of the conceptual invisibility of the passive smoker. A discourse stylistically motivated towards detachment was less able to 'see' the consequences of involvement. The 'discovery' of sidestream smoke created the capacity to see the previously unseeable and know the previously unknowable within the stylised boundaries of scientific cognition. Moreover, this stylistic ordering and reordering of reality reflects and reinforces a number of wider processual patterns, one of which has been illuminated by Frankenberg (Frankenberg, 1992).

Frankenberg describes the sick, in the history of epidemics, as a 'powerless other' and the well as a 'powerful same'. Having been identified, the former must go on to lose their 'otherness' and, in the interest of the latter, become the same as the 'same'. And following the development of sidestream smoke as scientific fact, this idea of a same and an other – a *social* sidestream and mainstream – characterised subsequent medical investigations of passive smoking and transformed its understanding of the phenomenon. These studies, commonly referred to as the 'spouse as index' studies (for example, Garfinkel (1981), Hirayama (1981) and Trichopolous *et al.* (1981)), examined morbidity and mortality rates amongst the spouses of tobacco smokers. They produced a range of results and provoked a variety of responses, but the important point for the purposes of this discussion is that the stylistic reordering of our social perceptions has been made. Whether one accepts that 'continued exposure to their husbands' smoking increased mortality from lung cancer in non-smokers up to two-fold' (Hirayama, 1981: 184) or one believes that the effect of passive smoking is 'at most quite small, if it exists at all' (Lee *et al.*, 1986: 104), our social 'sameness' or 'otherness' is stylistically defined. Moreover, it is done so at an individual level rather than a social one and, thus, the social forces that shape and underpin our social lives such as class and spatial location are marginalised. In claiming to see certain connections between previously discrete bodies and projecting those connections as privileged, then, medical science renders other possibilities unintelligible. Our 'sameness' or 'otherness' is represented as a matter of personal responsibility, a point central to the work of those writers involved in the critique of individualistic and victim blaming ideologies in health promotion discourse (Crawford, 1977; Graham, 1984).

To recap, I have argued, following Fleck, that medicine's understanding of tobacco as a threat to health involved more than a broadening of the medical knowledge base. Scientific knowledge is produced in relation to the possibilities of style rather than by accessing an external reality. The separation of tobacco smoke into chemical components and the reconstitution of those components into mainstream and sidestream smoke enabled medical science to ask a new set of questions about the relationship between tobacco and ill health and, ultimately, to produce new forms of knowledge about that relationship. Furthermore, I have argued that this stylistic ordering and reordering of reality can be mapped on to wider processual patterns and Frankenberg's images of the 'other' and the 'same' enabled us to interpret some of the relationships between this new scientific knowledge and those wider patterns of process. This culminated in the observation that our social connections and identities were being stylistically (mis)represented as individually controlled and directed. In the final section, I shall explore another set of mechanisms involved in the production of this privileged, new form of knowledge with a view, once again, to locating their emergence and development in style and process.

THE STYLISATION OF VISIBILITY

As we have noted, the reconstruction of tobacco smoke into a mainstream and a sidestream and the subsequent stylistic reordering of populations in terms of a 'same' and an 'other' encouraged medical science to ask new types of questions about the relationship between tobacco and ill health. No longer confined to the individual body, the health effects of tobacco smoking could now be traced through the stylised spaces and connections between bodies. Such thoughts encourage all bodies to come into the view of medical science. Indeed, no longer simply seen in terms of diseased/not diseased and, therefore, of differing interest to medicine, now all bodies are made visible for medical scrutiny. Moreover, it is a process that is grounded in the very procedures of medical investigation as well as its linguistic categories. One such procedure involves the utilisation of 'biochemical markers' as indicators of the extent to which non-smokers are exposed to environmental tobacco smoke. According to Lee (1988) the use of biochemical markers is a function of 'the possible unreliability of smoking habit information collected by self-report' (Lee, 1988: 13). For the purposes of this discussion, however, it also illuminates the way in which developments in scientific thinking and practice stylistically construct a world they purportedly reveal. Three groups of markers are commonly used, those based upon carbon monoxide, thiocyanate and nicotine (and its metabolite cotinine), and they are typically measured in samples of blood, urine and saliva. Lee questions the effectiveness of them all but, effective or otherwise, all are used to demonstrate the passive absorption of tobacco smoke by non-smokers. A number of points are of interest to us here. First, the use of biochemical markers promotes and legitimises the idea that bodies now 'reveal' the imprint of their connections with other bodies. No longer discrete and independent, bodies are now connected and interdependent. As we have seen, however, such knowledge is based upon the stylisation of our social identities rather than their revelation.

Second, since all bodies are embraced by the medical gaze – even in 'health' they are now the legitimate concern of medicine – they are all subject to the privileged readings of medical science. By its privileged readings of those bodies, science legitimates its claims based upon those readings – claims that, as Zola pointed out some time ago, extend the boundaries of medical involvement in our lives (Zola, 1972). For example, alongside the 'traditional' reasons for giving up smoking – 'I'll have less chance of getting lung cancer' – a recent No Smoking Day publication lists a number of others seemingly unrelated to bio-medical thought: 'I'll have more self-respect, I'll be more in control of my life' (No Smoking Day, 1994). Thus, life chances and self-respect become inseparable from health issues and both are promoted as individual concerns. Once again, the social forces that frame our lives and shape our identities are obscured, misrepresented in style.

Third, this notion of the stylisation of connections rather than their revelation is heightened by the actual scientific practices involved in the reading of biochemical markers. The presence of cotinine in urine, for example, is scientifically accepted as an accurate indication of nicotine absorption (Wald *et al.*, 1984; Greenberg *et al.*, 1991). However, nicotine is not in itself considered to be carcinogenic (Greenberg *et al.*, 1991). Its importance is based upon its relationship with other smoke constituents that are classified as carcinogenic. These remain hidden in the body and can only be rendered visible by way of association. However, as we have seen, those practices of association – enabling one set of properties to be identified in relation to another – are themselves implicated in the processes of knowledge production. Thus, visibility is produced rather than revealed; a new form of knowledge is made possible by shifts in a way of thinking, shifts intimately related to the notion of a social sidestream and, subsequently, to that of a reconstituted medical subject.

Finally, and in relation to the last point, the concept of biochemical markers not only stylistically 'marks out' the relationships between bodies, it is also involved in a process of 'marking out' a new set of possibilities concerning the health of those bodies. For example, in an analysis of the body in consumer culture, Featherstone argues that an increasing 'emphasis upon body maintenance and appearance . . . suggests two basic categories: the inner body and the outer body' (Featherstone, 1991a: 171). The former articulates concerns about the functioning and maintenance of the body; the latter embraces ideas, amongst others, about its appearance and presentation. Within consumer culture, he continues, the two 'become conjoined': 'the prime purpose of the maintenance of the inner body becomes the enhancement of the outer body' (Featherstone, 1991a: 171).

Without wishing to pursue the point too far, then, one might see the stylistic marking of the inner body as part of a process that also maps out a series of implications for the outer body. Indeed, in much the same way as No Smoking Day promoted enhanced life chances and self-respect as benefits of abstaining from tobacco smoking, so the Health Education Authority promotes aesthetic gains: 'You'll smell fresher. No more bad breath or stained fingers or teeth. You'll be nicer to be with. Remember the slogan kiss a non-smoker and taste the difference' (Health Education Authority, 1991b: 2–3). Thus, notions of social attractiveness become 'conjoined' with bio-medical issues; the aesthetic becomes 'marked out' in relation to the new facts of science.

It is the argument of this chapter, then, that whilst we are being encouraged to think differently about the relationship between tobacco and ill health, we are not encouraged to think differently about the scientific facts underpinning and legitimating this conceptual shift. Informed by Fleck's idea that scientific knowledge is produced in relation to the possibilities of stylised thought, this essay offers a constructionist account of this process, an account which examines in detail some of the mechanisms involved in the emergence and development of passive smoking as scientific fact.

It has been suggested that one of the most significant of those mechanisms involves the idea that a cigarette generates two types of smoke. Thus, in relation to a particular cultural style of thought that deconstructs and reconstructs the phenomena of its investigations, the reduction of tobacco smoke to its chemical components and the reconstitution of those parts into mainstream and sidestream smoke provoked medical science to ask a new set of questions about the relationship between tobacco and ill health. Those questions then made it possible for medicine to conceptualise the effects of tobacco beyond the individual body and rendered the previously invisible passive smoker visible to medical scrutiny. Furthermore, it was suggested that these stylistic developments could be mapped on to deeper processual patterns, notably those identified by Frankenberg's images of the 'other' and the 'same' and that the ideas and practices associated with biochemical markers, marking out the body in the cultural terms of medical science, also marked out our conceptions of our sameness/otherness in terms of our perceptions of the social body and our place in it. This was then extended to incorporate a brief discussion of the changing nature of health, in which the 'legitimate' aesthetic appearance of the outer body was seen to be being marked out in conjunction with the stylised representation of the inner body.

NOTE

1 This chapter draws upon some material discussed at greater length in Jackson (1994).

Chapter 10

Accidents and the risk society

Some problems with prevention

Judith Green

INTRODUCTION

Accident prevention has become a key area for health promotion, with recent policy initiatives recommending educational interventions to reduce accident rates. Such strategies have had little documented success. This chapter first examines how 'lay' views of accidents are constructed in professional accounts as the problem to be overcome in achieving successful accident prevention. Second, it explores lay and professional accounts through data from an exploratory study of how we construct the accidental in everyday life. These accounts suggest some explanations of the failure of accident prevention.

RISK AND ACCIDENT PREVENTION

Risk has become somewhat of an obsession in sociology of late, and calculation of risk has been seen as a key characteristic of modern life. In his analysis of the implications of modern high risk technologies, for instance, Beck (1992a; 1992b) claims that we are no longer primarily divided by access to wealth, but by our relative susceptibility to risk. For Giddens risk is the dominant organising principle in contemporary culture: 'To live in the universe of high modernity is to live in an environment of chance and risk ... Fate and destiny have no part to play in such a system' (Giddens, 1991: 109).

Castel further argues that discourses of risk have emerged as the technique by which prevention has been made possible as a strategy (Castel, 1991). This focus on the role of risk calculation and its implications for how we perceive fate and destiny seems a useful point of departure for an analysis of current policy in accident prevention. If we can take Giddens' statement as a workable summary of aspects of contemporary discourse, or at least the cluster of beliefs that relate to causality and legitimate ways of imputing it, we find that the accident, as it is conventionally constructed by accident prevention literature, has no place.

What are accidents? In everyday usage, the label 'accident' is used for a large and seemingly disparate range of events. A list of such events might include an industrial injury, an unintended pregnancy, incontinence in children, a broken plate and a car crash. Little unites the outcomes of these events, but they are grouped together by assumptions about their cause. An accident, ideally, is characterised by lack of intention (no one meant it to happen) and by unpredictability (no one knew it was going to happen just then). An accident is apparently something that happens 'out of the blue' that no one can be blamed for.

Health promotion is largely concerned with a particular subset of the misfortunes we label as accidental: those that result in a recognisable injury. These injuries cause a considerable amount of death, disability and distress and the risk factors for them have been the subject of increasing study since the middle of the twentieth century. In recent years national and international policy initiatives have encouraged research into accident rates and interventions to try to reduce those rates. In 1985 the World Health Organisation set a target for reducing accident mortality in Europe by 25 per cent by the year 2000, by concentrating specifically on home, road and occupational accidents (WHO, 1985). Given that this target was likely to be surpassed in Britain, the Department of Health's (1992a) strategy document *The Health of the Nation* set new targets:

A. To reduce the death rate for accidents among children aged under 15 by at least 33% by 2005 (from 6.7 per 100,000 population in 1990 to no more than 4.5 per 100,000).
B. To reduce the death rate for accidents among young people aged 15–24 by at least 25% by 2005 (from 24.0 per 100,000 population to no more than 18.0 per 100,000).
C. To reduce the death rate for accidents among people aged 65 and over by at least 33% by 2005 (from 56.7 per 100,000 population to no more than 38 per 100,000).

(Department of Health, 1992a: 104)

Health promotion operates within a discourse of risk and its management in which the accident, as a random misfortune over which one can have no control, has no obvious place. The accident becomes something other than the unforeseen outcome of coincidence or fate. As epidemiology maps an ever-increasing range of risk factors for accidental injury and their social distribution becomes more exactly known, the accident becomes patterned and predictable. Having an accident results no longer from fate but from ignorance, miscalculation or the deliberate negligence of known risks. Accidents, in short, should no longer happen.

MOUNTAIN ACCIDENTS – AN EXAMPLE

The annual statistics produced by the Lake District Search and Mountain Rescue Association (LDSAMRA, 1992) provide an initial example of this contemporary view of accidents as constructed through an analysis of risks. The annual report describes 255 cases of 'Mountain accidents' which occurred in 1991. For each case, details of the type, site and outcomes of the accident, prevailing weather conditions and the time of the call-out are listed. In addition details relating to the victim are given: demographic information, the type of clothing they were wearing, the equipment they carried, and an assessment of their experience. Examples include falls while walking and climbing as well as rescues of those suffering from hypothermia after becoming lost or benighted.

One implication of these data is that there are two levels of cause for each of these misfortunes. First is the immediate cause, for instance, slipping on a wet path or collapse. But before this were the conditions that made such an event more likely, such as the environmental and other factors that can be used to predict 'an accident waiting to happen'. Thus the inadequacy of a walker's clothing is noted, or their lack of experience. Victims miscalculate risks by underestimating the weather; they flout safety by wearing inappropriate shoes and clothing and they display ignorance of risks in their lack of experience. Interestingly, responsibility is not inferred from any causal link between the miscalculation of specific risk and the particular injury sustained. Ignoring or miscalculating risks such as weather or inadequate clothing implies somehow a more general culpability. In one case, for instance, a man suffers spinal injuries and a fractured scapula in circumstances that do not appear to require any particular precautions. His accident happens thus: 'On walk from car park to pose for a photograph, fell backwards over a boulder' (LDSAMRA, 1992: Case 208). It is still noted that his clothing consisted of 'canvas shoes, town clothes' and that his experience was 'doubtful'.

Luck, it seems, has been evaporated in this environment of known (or at least knowable) risks. Indeed it is mentioned only in the context of avoiding the consequences of negligent action. In one case (LDSAMRA, 1992: Case 24), for instance, a man who was solo climbing fell 500 feet and sustained a sprained neck and lacerations to scalp and nose. The outcome was described as 'very lucky' in parentheses, which it may well have been, but there is no suggestion that any of those who suffered accidents may have been 'unlucky' in that it happened to them. Indeed the public information at the end of the report (see Figure 10.1) explicitly holds the victim responsible. 'British mountains can be killers', it notes, 'if proper care is not taken' (LDSAMRA, 1992: 66). If proper care is taken (a daunting prospect involving predicting not only the weather and the physical environment but also protecting against what the recommendations call 'plain damned carelessness') accidents should not happen.

HEALTH PROMOTION: THE REPORTED CONFLICT BETWEEN LAY AND PROFESSIONAL VIEWS

These two strands of risk and preventability resonate with the key concerns of contemporary health promotion. There is a professional voice in the literature on accident prevention that constructs as a foil a contrasting 'lay' voice. The professional construction of accidents (as predictable from known risk factors) engages in a constant dialogue with an off-stage 'lay' construction, which is reported to stress fate and therefore unpredictability. The lay view is presented as only looking at the individual event. This leads, it is implied, to a misguided and anachronistic view of accidents as unpredictable and therefore unpreventable. For health promotion, these lay beliefs form a barrier to be overcome in the campaign to reduce accidents. This can only be achieved if the individual misfortunes that we call 'accidents' are seen as part of a rate – as part of a larger pattern which makes sense.

Here are just a few examples of how this debate is presented in the literature:

> Accidents are not totally random events striking innocent victims like bolts from the blue, although they are often described in this way. Accidents have a natural history in which predisposing factors converge to produce an accidental event.
>
> (Stone, 1991: 61)

> It is vital to counter the view of accidents as random events due to bad luck.
>
> (Henwood, 1992: 26)

A handbook produced for health workers by the Child Accident Prevention Trust notes the 'common-sense' usage of the term accident relating to ideas of chance and premeditation, but says that accidents are on the whole predictable events and 'there is a base for intervention and preventive action' (CAPT, 1989). At its least compromising, the professional view completely dissolves the accident:

> Nearly all 'accidents' contain an element of neglect by exposure to risk, except those accidents which are true acts of God. Some would argue that these too can be avoided by appropriate action.
>
> (Polnay, 1992: 105)

There is, then, a professional orthodoxy that all accidents are preventable, and that it is necessary to educate the public to abandon fatalistic views

LIVE A LITTLE LONGER

British mountains can be killers if proper care is not taken. The following notes cover the minimum precautions if you want to avoid getting hurt or lost, and so inconveniencing or endangering others as well as your-selves.

Clothing
This could be colourful, warm, windproof and waterproof. Wear boots with nails or moulded rubber soles, not shoes, plimsolls, or gum-boots. Take a woollen cap and a spare jersey; it is always colder on the tops.

Food
In addition to the usual sandwiches, take chocolate, dates, mint cake or similar sweet things which restore energy quickly. If you don't need them yourself, someone else may.

Equipment
This must include map, compass, and at least one reliable watch in the party. A whistle, torch and spare batteries and bulbs (six blasts or flashes repeated at minute intervals signal an emergency), and, in winter conditons, an ice-axe and survival bag are essential. Climbers are all urged to wear helmets.

Company
Don't go alone, and make sure party leaders are experienced. Take special care of the youngest and weakest in dangerous places.

Emergencies
Don't press on if conditions are against you – turn back even if it upsets your plan. Learn first aid, and keep injured or exhausted people warm until help reaches you. Get a message to the Police for help as soon as possible, and report changes of route or time-table to them if someone is expecting you. The Police will do the rest.

Dangers Which Can Always Be Avoided
and should be until you know how to cope with them:
Precipices
  Slopes of ice,
    or steep snow,
      or very steep grass (especially frozen),
        or unstable boulders.
Gullies and stream beds.
Streams in spate.
Snow cornices on ridges or gully tops.
  Over-ambition.
    Plain damned carelessness.

Dangers Which May Surprise You
and should be guarded against:
Weather changes – mist, gale, rain or snow.
Get forecasts, and watch the sky in all quarters.

Ice on paths

**Carry an ice-axe and crampons
know how to use them.**

Excessive cold or heat.

Dress sensibly, and take a spare jersey.

Incipient exhaustion.

Know the signs; rest and keep warm.

Accident or illness.

Don't panic. If you send for help, make sure that the rescuers know exactly where to come.

Flight of time.

**Learn your own pace. Plan your walk.
Allow double time in winter conditions.**

It is no disgrace to turn back if you are not certain.
A party must be governed by the capabilities of the weakest member.

Figure 10.1 'Live a Little Longer'
Source: Lake District Search and Rescue Association, 1992

which hold them to be otherwise. Given that accidents are constructed as essentially preventable events, it may be useful to look at the range of strategies proposed to prevent them before examining the success of these strategies.

Conventionally, the main accident prevention strategies are divided into the '3 Es': education, engineering and enforcement (see, for instance, Cliff (1984)). Education involves raising awareness of risks and how to avoid them. Examples might include road safety training for children or leaflets about hazards in the home. Engineering refers to changing the environment to either reduce the risk of an accident happening or to reduce the damage of an accident that does happen. The development of flameproof material for nightdresses and child-resistant aspirin tops are engineering interventions. Enforcement involves introducing legal sanctions against behaviour likely to either cause accidents or increase the risk of damage from accidents, such as legislation making wearing helmets compulsory for riding a motorbike.

This obviously gives much scope for preventative action, and *The Health of the Nation* (Department of Health, 1992a) has suggestions for achieving targets that fall into all three categories. There is some evidence that both engineering and enforcement strategies can reduce the mortality rates from specific hazards. The introduction of legislation to enforce seat belt use for drivers and front seat passengers in Britain in 1983 is one example of an 'enforcement' strategy that achieved the aim of reducing mortality and serious injury to drivers (Department of Transport, 1985). Engineering approaches have also had some documented successes. The introduction of flameproof material for nightdresses and the child-resistant pill bottle tops reduced mortality rates in childhood from burns and poisoning respectively (Croft and Sibert, 1992) and changes to road layouts to separate pedestrians from motorised traffic have been shown to reduce childhood road traffic accidents (Sutherland, 1992). The 'Children can't fly' campaign in New York, which distributed free window guards for families with pre-school children, significantly reduced the mortality from falls from windows (Spiegel and Lindaman, 1977).

In contrast, there has been paltry evidence that educational interventions affect accident rates (Croft and Sibert, 1992). Despite this, they are the most commonly used and advocated strategies. One review of accident prevention interventions found that the majority were those designed to raise awareness or increase knowledge (Popay and Young, 1993). *The Health of the Nation* shared the preference for educational interventions, noting: 'the government will rely primarily on information and education and will avoid the imposition of unnecessary regulations' (Department of Health, 1992a: 106).

Research provides few grounds for optimism about the likely success of such approaches. One study of accidents to children (Carter and Jones,

1993), for instance, found no significant differences in either knowledge about safety or even in ownership of safety equipment between parents of children who had had accidents and those who had not. The authors still concluded that what was needed was 'more education', opportunistically at the child health surveillance clinic and during home visits. Melia *et al.* (1989) studied the homes of children who had reported an accident to hospital and a group of matched controls. Although they found that those who had had accidents were more likely to have fathers who were unemployed and have had an upset at home over the last twelve months, there was no significant difference in the number of safety hazards spotted by health visitors in the homes of the two groups of children. Hazards were the unsafe practices that are the target of much health promotion aimed at parents: absence of fire-guards, loose flexes, access to matches, windows openable by children and loose stair carpets.

Despite such findings, education continues to be offered as a universal panacea for reducing the number of accidents. One paper on accidents to the elderly noted the complex chain of causation of accidents, concluding that: 'We had difficulty attributing an event to any one factor. Most resulted from an interaction of environmental hazards, physical disability, and carelessness or excessive risk taking' (Graham and Firth, 1992: 32). However, the authors still suggested that the key question for accident prevention was 'whether an education programme for the whole elderly population or specific targeting of selected patients would be more effective in reducing home accidents?' (Graham and Firth, 1992: 32).

In this epidemiological research, the implication is that the failure of educational initiatives and prevention policies (or at least their lack of documented success) is attributable to the persistence of lay beliefs that hold accidents to be unpredictable and therefore unpreventable. Sociology has been more concerned with the structural barriers to prevention.

Roberts and her co-workers (Roberts *et al.*, 1992; 1993), for instance, in their work on safety on a Glasgow housing estate, suggested a structural critique of accident prevention strategies. They found that although professionals adopted a model which held accidents to be caused by negligence and believed that more education was needed, parents were actually well aware of risks, in fact more aware of specific local dangers than professionals. They took a considerable range of actions, both individually and as campaigners, to keep their children safe, and of course managed to do so almost all of the time. Education aimed at increasing awareness of dangers merely tends to increase maternal anxiety as hazards were often environmental ones that little could be done about by individual carers: sockets with no on/off switches, balcony railings which toddlers could crawl under and unguarded holes left by workers. In addition to the physical dangers of the environment, the sheer cost of providing all the recommended safety equipment to prevent home accidents was prohibitive for families on low incomes.

Such a structural critique implies one explanation for the persistence of educational strategies despite their lack of success: that they focus attention away from the structural inequalities which pattern accident rates and utilise what Crawford (1986) has called a 'victim blaming' ideology. This explanation has received some attention from Tombs (1991), in his analysis of ideologies of 'accident prone workers' in the chemical industry, and from Naidoo (1986: 25–6) in her comment on the individualistic ideologies of media campaigns to promote home safety, which ignore the social distribution of accident risks and mitigate against collective action.

IS THERE A DIFFERENCE BETWEEN LAY AND PROFESSIONAL PERSPECTIVES?

Such structural critiques offer a convincing account of the persistence of education as the key strategy of health promotion, despite the lack of demonstrated success. Here, I would like to argue that there is perhaps a more fundamental tension at the heart of the idea of accident prevention that makes failure predictable. This tension is not, as has been suggested by the literature, between 'lay' and 'professional' beliefs, but rather lies within our ideas of the accidental itself. First, although lay beliefs are presented as being about the unpredictability and lack of blameworthiness of accidents, even the most cursory look at what people say about accidents reflects more ambiguity than this, as is apparent in colloquialisms such as 'it was an accident waiting to happen', 'accidents will happen' and the ironic 'we could arrange for you to have an accident'. Such folk wisdom implicitly acknowledges that accidents are both random, unpredictable events on an individual level, but patterned and predictable at a statistical level. The remainder of this chapter explores this tension using some data from a pilot study on how accidents are constructed as a category of misfortune. The way in which accidental happenings are described and debated suggests far more complexity in our ideas about accidents than the mere persistence of beliefs in fate and luck.

The data used are from interviews with people chosen for their expertise on some aspect of accidents. Many people in modern life have some formal or legitimate role in the monitoring, analysis or prevention of accidents. Six of these interviews were with people who identified themselves as having some professional concern with accidents or their prevention. They were an actuary, an astrologer (with a particular interest in the astrology of accidents), an RAF doctor, two Home Accident clerks (who are the people responsible for collecting statistics as part of the Department of Trade and Industry's Home Accident Surveillance System) and a health visitor. Five interviews were with groups of children aged between 5 and 11, who are the major subjects of much accident prevention, and thus key 'lay' people. All interviews were audio-taped and transcribed. The following is based on an analysis of these transcripts.

WHAT PEOPLE SAY ABOUT ACCIDENTS

First, all of those interviewed, whether 'lay' people, like the children, or 'professionals', like the actuary whose work perhaps epitomises the modern mapping of risk, readily identified the kind of event that they would label 'an accident'. They provided definitions which appeared to coincide with the 'lay view' that emerged from the accident prevention literature. They all, in summary, could provide a general definition of an accident which stressed the unpredictability or the blamelessness of the act:

> 'An accident is something that goes wrong . . . by accident that actually hurts you' (Amelia, age 8).

> 'Things like electrocuted yourself by accident . . . you can't predict that' (Actuary).

> 'An accident for me is a bodily mishap that happens to people without any intention of hurt, either on the part of the sufferer or the agent' (Astrologer).

> 'It's people falling down the stairs, breaking plates in the sink . . . half the time when you ask a question how they done it, they've just tripped for no apparent reason' (Home Accident Clerk 1).

> 'It's a coincidence, like. Some people get accidents and some don't' (Leroy, age 10).

However, it soon becomes clear that these initial working definitions only serve for ideal or hypothetical cases. When people begin to talk about actual events, they described accidents as neither unambiguously unpredictable nor unambiguously morally neutral.

Unpredictability

First, specific accidents may not be unpredictable: some may appear to be inevitable, as Amelia and Jessica note:

> Amelia (age 8):   'Some of them are going to happen anyway.'
> Jessica (age 6):   'Yeah, because there might be a bomb and it's got to blow up.'

The actuary talked about accidents first as specific events, which could not be predicted and which would, as he put it, 'come out as a sort of blip' in the statistics. But in this respect they were like any of the other uncertainties that he dealt with, and would be averaged out:

'They [life assurance firms] might look at the stats on accidental death and say 'are they significant?' If... they were getting a significant number of accidental deaths they would have to [load the premiums] but typically it's the case that things even themselves out' (Actuary).

For him, however carefully the rates of events (be they accidents or any other misfortune) were mapped, you could still not predict any individual event:

'This guy ... might look as healthy as can be, a good risk, and then he just pops his clogs' (Actuary).

This contrast between the predictable and unpredictable is presented in epidemiological terms by this professional: the argument that population statistics are not very useful for predicting what is going to happen to a particular individual. Other respondents also made a distinction between the predictable and the unpredictable, though, even if not in these epidemiological terms. They talked about different classes of event rather than different levels of measurement.

One of the home accident clerks, for instance, thought that accidents could be divided into two kinds, those that could be prevented because the causes were known:

'I mean most of it is carelessness, but if people could be made more aware perhaps they would, you know, like they've got curly flexes for kettles and so on' (Home Accident Clerk 1),

and those about which nothing could be done because they were genuinely random occurrences that were not predictable:

'Some, as I say, I suppose what I call the sensible accidents can be helped. But as I say the children falling from swings, you'll never stop will you?' (Home Accident Clerk 1).

Her colleague likewise initially attributed half of the accidents she saw to:

'Stupidity really, carelessness, which half of the accidents come from' (Home Accident Clerk 2),

and the other half as 'proper' accidents, which could not be prevented: 'They just happen' (Home Accident Clerk 2). Even these remaining 'ideal' accidents were not, though, purely random occurrences. First, the idea of the 'accident prone' individual serves to reduce the unpredictability:

'My eldest one is always falling down the stairs, always rushing about. I bet she falls down the stairs once a week, honestly. 'Cause she's erratic mainly. There's nothing wrong with the stair carpet, it doesn't matter whether she's got boots or slippers on' (Home Accident Clerk 2).

Second, other agents, such as local councils who failed to maintain uneven pavements, or the unsafe conditions of local bed and breakfast accommodation for young families, were mentioned as contributing to the conditions that made such accidents more likely. Such agents, as well as the victim, may also be held culpable in the final analysis of the event. Blamelessness, like unpredictability, only described accidents in general. Particular accidents were the subject of considerable moral enquiry.

Moral Neutrality

The label 'accident' is awarded only provisionally, and seems to designate an event within the legitimate arena of moral negotiation. It is also a label which is constructed through a process of such negotiation. This negotiation is reported to first be with oneself, for negligence:

'When [daughter] caught her finger in the train door, I thought "why did we sit in that part of the carriage" – the door slammed and that was her finger . . . you do feel quite guilty and that – I really thought it was my fault I'd sat her there' (Home Accident Clerk 2).

'I was on a step ladder and thought I was on a stool . . . and went to step off and I was four feet in the air instead of two feet . . . It was my fault – stupid, careless!' (Home Accident Clerk 1).

Although one might refer to such events as 'accidents' they are clearly not purely blameless events. Only accidents in general could be described as 'no one's fault' and most specific instances could be traced to particular causes, with blame potentially attaching either to the victim or another for negligence. The actuary, for instance, suggested Acts of God as classic accidents, but when asked to think of instances, could only identify being struck by lightning:

'being hit by lightning or something like that, or being drowned at sea would count – or it might do . . . but it wouldn't be an act of God, it would be an act of negligence on the part of the ship's captain' (Actuary).

Similarly, he said, most traffic accidents would involve some human agency:

'they're a crap driver [or] if their brakes fail, it's the fault of the mechanic who serviced their car' (Actuary).

It is apparent that there are no events that are unambiguously accidental in terms of the definitions first suggested – the term emerges as a provisional category only, and one which is open to negotiation. Indeed, in conversations with children, it seems that stories about accidents serve specifically to organise and debate ideas about moral responsibility:

Maria (age 8):   'We was sliding down the stairs and I was on her lap and then suddenly I fell down and she fell on top of me.'
Anja (age 6):   'And I bumped my head and it really hurt!'
JG: 'And was that an accident?'
Maria: 'Well it was an accident 'cause we were never told that it would hurt us.'

The following excerpt refers to an incident that was related to me by several of the children. The incident involved a boy (whose identity changed in the different performances of the story) who falls from a pole in the playground, injuring himself seriously enough to need hospital attention. Amelia is telling the story with Jessica's help:

Amelia (age 8):   'People go round that pole sometimes and lots of people climb up and he climbed the pole and he slipped . . . but I wouldn't really say that was an accident.'
JG: 'You wouldn't? Why not?'
Amelia: 'Well, I don't think it was his actual fault because someone had done it before I think, and told him to do it – said like "I dare you". I don't think it was his fault, but . . .'
Jessica (age 6):   '. . . he shouldn't have done it.'
Amelia: 'He shouldn't have done it, anyway.'

Children of course learn early on how to manipulate these ambiguities over responsibility and blame. This can be simply to avoid blame, as Anja confesses: 'I hit Zara once, but I said "it was an accident" (Anja, age 6), but also for humorous effect. Richard is one of a group of boys who were busy squashing ants with their fists on the table as I talked to them:

'Like that was an accident – I just tried to stop Leroy killing one, and then my hand accidentally went "crash"! (Richard, age 8).

Adults who did not seem to recognise the ambiguities of culpability and responsibility could be frustrating, as Jessica notes:

Jessica (age 6):   'Once Hanifa [class teacher] was chatting with

Yesim, because she [Yesim] had hurt her hand, it was cut right there ... and she was saying "was it an accident or was it on purpose?" and Yesim said "I don't know" and Hanifa said "You must know if it was an accident or on purpose" and Yesim said "I don't know" and Hanifa said "just tell me".'

JG: 'Do you think you always do know whether ...'

Jessica: 'No, but Hanifa thought you must ...'

Sometimes these ambiguities were followed through to their logical conclusion, and respondents could not think of any actual events that would count as ideal, blameless accidents. The RAF doctor, asked what kind of accidents might happen in training, points to the difficulty of finding a specific event that matches the ideal definition of an accident:

'Let me think of a case. You fly into a hill in cloud, which is always down to pilot error really because he didn't recognise the weather was bad and abort early enough and get up to a higher level' (RAF doctor).

All such events would be investigated by a board.

JG: 'Does the board ever find it was an accident? Do accidents ever happen?'

RAF Doctor: 'I mean basically it can be a mechanical error or a pilot error. There's only two things that can go wrong really, I suppose. The aeroplane or the pilot.'

We might suppose that even if such an event had to be officially designated a 'cause' then it would still be unofficially described as a tragic accident. However, the doctor went on to describe a mess room ritual that would happen in the event of a pilot dying in such a crash. This involves, among other things, a ritualistic rubbishing of the dead pilot's professional reputation:

'People start talking about memories of him, and the memories tend to be, "oh well, he always did take risks", you know, "you know what he was like he always pushed it" ' (RAF doctor).

The notion that an accident could happen to any one in mid-air is perhaps too much for anyone expected to get into a plane every day and fly to cope with. Such misfortunes have to be explained as predictable – and therefore preventable – events.

PREVENTION

If this group of people, both in their professional and lay roles, agreed that accidents could, at least in theory, be prevented, how did they think this could be done? When I asked children about if and how we can stop accidents happening, they could repeat safety advice they had learnt at school, often as a kind of mantra:

JG: 'Some of you had some ideas about how you could stop accidents happening . . .'

All in chorus
(six boys aged 6 to 11): 'Look, listen, learn . . .'

Matthew (age 6): 'Stay in your bedroom . . .'

Several
[laughs, loud noises of protest]: 'Stupid!'

JG: 'So how do you stop accidents happening?'

Amelia (age 8): 'Be very, very, careful.'

The adults provided advice that was broadly consistent with the children's accounts of carefulness as the first line of defence:

'With tiny children it [safety] has to be your first priority – you can't be too careful' (Health Visitor).

JG: 'So can you prevent accidents happening?'

Accident Clerk: 'Yes, by being more careful . . .'

Accidents could be prevented if enough care was taken to reduce risks. However, again, this advice was given in a general sense, and often individual accidents were seen as rather more complex in their causation – or at least the risk calculation involved in preventing them in practice was seen as being somewhat impractical. Simon, for instance, points to the limitations of Sam's advice on accident prevention in the kitchen:

Simon (age 10): 'When I was drying up . . . [I was] trying to dry it too fast, and the plate slipped out of my hand, and I got grounded for a week. And I didn't think that was fair . . .'

Matthew (age 9): 'Yeah, and like Sam said . . . "well you should have been holding it with two hands!" '

Simon: 'Well, if I'd been holding it in two hands I wouldn't have been able to dry up, so Sam's a bit wrong!'

The other practical limitation to the operation of safety advice was the empirical evidence that it could sometimes be ignored with impunity:

JG: 'So are there some people who have more accidents than others?'

Leroy (age 10): 'Like I've never had an accident before . . .'

Matthew (age 9): 'But he was sitting on the chair right . . . with two legs up like that – and he could have fallen back and broken his leg!'

When pushed to describe how individual accidents could be avoided, children were quick to point to flaws in 'safety first' logic:

Jessica (age 6):   '[You could prevent] falling off your bike, because someone could be there to catch you.'

Amelia (age 8):   '[laughs] I know, but someone might not be there! ... I was just riding along and I knew I was going too fast and I just pulled on my front brake and the back wheel went [makes noise] and I went flying over' [demonstrates].

JG: 'So whose fault was that?'

Amelia: 'I don't think it was anyone's fault, do you? The people who put the tarmac there!' [laughs].

Safety advice, it appears, is not particularly useful for preventing specific accidental events. The children's recitation of 'look, listen, learn' suggests another role for safety advice, though. Precautions (be they wearing proper clothing for mountain walking or fixing cooker guards in the home) seem to have little causal relationship with specific accident events, either in research on accidents or in people's accounts of the causes of accidents. They do, however, demonstrate an adherence to the *concept* of prevention. The health visitor, for instance, describes how she burnt her leg on holiday:

'We're on this tiny little motorbike up a mountain – we had a helmet, would you believe – we were the only people in Kos to have a helmet! [laughs], so we took that precaution – but we were wearing only shorts ... I'd didn't think it would burn me' (Health Visitor).

When they are taken up, precautions are employed as *talismans* against misfortune, rather than as rational or instrumental attempts to reduce specific risk. Wearing a cycle safety helmet or providing a stair gate makes us feel safer not merely because it reduces in any causal way the likelihood of a head injury or a fall downstairs – but because it demonstrates that we did all we could, that we respected the calculability of risk.

DISCUSSION

Both professional and lay people describe particular events as 'accidents' and utilise a working definition of 'ideal type' accidents which suggests that they are unpredictable and unwilled. Such definitions are tenuous, though; describing an event as an 'accident' is only a provisional explanation, pending more detailed investigation of the specific features of a case. This is clear in these everyday stories of accidents described above, in which events are analysed for precipitating factors and possible culpability. The tension between the accident as a random misfortune and the accident as a predictable outcome of known risks is not one between lay and professional accounts. Both lay and professional accounts are inherently paradoxical, in two senses. The first is that the ideal accident is constructed as a blameless event, yet in practice accidents are the subject of considerable debate about responsibility and culpability. There are few specific events that fulfil the criteria of ideal accidents.

Second, to define an event as an 'accident' relies on what are seen to be premodern beliefs (in fate, chance or *fortuna*), yet accidents can only exist within a modern, rationalist cosmology, in which there are known causes for most events and what is 'left over' gets defined as accidental. Accidents are the remnants of our classificatory system, defined not by their outcomes, but by what they are not. An event is accidental not because of any innate characteristics, but because it is *not* something else (a suicide, vandalism, child abuse). Inevitably, such definitions are provisional, since some other future verdict cannot be precluded and the designation is always, potentially if not overtly, in dispute. Even the coroner's officially 'final' verdict on a fatal accident, itself the result of a moral interrogation (Green, 1992a), can be the subject of further public and private debate about whether 'accident' was indeed the appropriate classification. It seems that such a category of left-over events is a necessary one as there will always be (in our classification of misfortunes) some events that we cannot explain in terms of predictability or moral intent.

If this perhaps suggests that accidents will not stop happening because there is a need for such a category, it does not explain why specific interventions fail to prevent specific accidents. Castel (1991) has suggested that one feature of risk factors is that they are potentially limitless. In terms of accident prevention, we can certainly produce ever more sophisticated accounts of the risks for accidents: socio-demographic factors, psychological attributes, occupation, leisure pursuits, equipment design faults, etc. There is clearly a tension, though, between what we know to be risk factors at the population level and the logical impossibility of translating that population risk into an individual preventative action. This is not a problem of lay people failing to understand the patterned nature of accidents. Both professionals and lay people recognised this tension, and it seemed that engaging in accident prevention was an activity designed somehow to manage this. In short, preventative actions were taken not in an instrumental way to reduce personal accident risks, but as ritual actions to demonstrate an awareness of population risks.

There is perhaps a search for meaning for all misfortune at the individual level, where a statistical explanation of risk factors will not suffice. The accidental provides a provisional explanation for that which is at the limits of rational explanation. Public health departments have been charged with the thankless task of reducing accident rates through educational strategies. They may succeed in reducing injury and fatality rates for specific types of injuries, although Roberts and others (Roberts *et al.*, 1993) have pointed to some structural limitations to the likely success of this project. There will also presumably always be a category of events that lie outside current explanatory categories – the remnants of our classification systems that we provisionally call accidents. Events may be predictable on a statistical level; accidents are not. Accidents may prove rather difficult to prevent.

CONCLUSION

In conclusion, I have argued that in part health promotion has engaged with a straw person in its presentation of the 'lay' view of accidents. When we come to look at this view, it is not so different from the professional view, in that it too is paradoxical. First there is no such thing as an ideal accident, the 'bolt from the blue' which is a purely blameless event. All actual accidents are labelled as such merely provisionally and as part of a process of moral negotiation. Second, there is a tension between accidents as constructed by an epidemiological mapping of their risk factors and accidents as they are experienced by individuals. Accident prevention is problematic as a strategy for reducing accident rates, but does seem to have some force as a ritual activity by which we construct ourselves as part of the risk society.

ACKNOWLEDGEMENTS

I am grateful to David Armstrong and Nicki Thorogood, who provided helpful advice on earlier drafts of this paper.

Chapter 11

Chance and modernity
Accidents as a public health problem

Lindsay Prior

CHANCE AND MODERNITY

In his *The Taming of Chance* Ian Hacking (1990) locates the decade
around 1660 as the birthtime of probability – the point at which chance
was tamed. From then onward, one might say, the capriciousness of
events was overcome, and almost all types of occurrence were reinter-
preted so as to make them appear calculable and predictable. Naturally,
the first forms of chance to be precisely tamed were the games of chance
(Hacking, 1975). So whereas, for example, in the early modern world the
fall of the dice and the choice of a playing card were things that appeared
to be unpredictable and random in every sense of the word, during the
late seventeenth and early eighteenth centuries such events came to be
regarded as predictable and calculable ones. Thus, the probability of
throwing two consecutive sixes with one die came to be calculated as
1/36. And the probability of, say, drawing a playing card with a face value
of less than five from a full pack as 4/13.

This linking of the mathematical concepts of probability with games of
chance eventually overflowed into more serious considerations – including
of course the calculation of the chances of life and death themselves.
(And what could be more serious than that?) Though as Hald (1990)
points out, even in considerations of the life table, the symbols of games
of chance were still applied. Thus Christian Huygens (1629–95), who
seems to have been the first mathematician to apply a probabilistic interpretation to the life table, still tended to consider such tables in terms of
the image of a lottery with a 100 tickets. And following Huygens, numerous other mathematicians improved upon the basic actuarial themes. Thus
de Moivre (1667–1754), for example, calculated the separate probabilities
of life and death for males and females in different age intervals. He also
published the first textbook on insurance mathematics and, rather like
many of the other mathematicians during this period, generally sought to
rid the world of the 'superstition' that there is any such thing as 'Luck'
(Hald, 1990: 406).

These various mathematical deliberations were, of course, eventually absorbed into numerous forms of professional practice. Most important of all, the new concepts of probability were called upon to support that most rational of all the organisational expressions of modern capitalism – namely, industrial systems of insurance assessment. Later, they also formed the basis of numerous technical styles of social assessment such as those involved in what we now refer to as epidemiology. And these social uses of mathematics are perhaps the most significant from our point of view, for it was they that were above all responsible for the construction of an actuarial vision of human existence: a vision in which the very chances of living *per se* were seen to be calculable and precisely assessable events. In that respect, we might say that William Farr's *English Life Table Number One* (1843) expresses, better than almost anything else, that aspect of modern consciousnessthat regards the unfathomable secrets of human mortality as in some way controllable, and rationally 'accountable'. Moreover, and in terms of a wider perspective, we can also see that such ways of looking at empirical reality were merely one among many kindred visions in which the social world was, as Condorcet (1743–94) was to argue, a 'grandiose geometrical construction' (Picavet, 1971: 110) in which everything occurred according to identifiable causes: a world in which there was nothing accidental and nothing unexpected; a world in which everything could be accounted for in terms of a social calculus. (A more recent expression of this enlightenment vision is presented by Dawkins (1988), when he reduces 'miracles' and the miraculous to improbable but nevertheless calculable events.)

In short, then, it would seem that from the eighteenth century onward the apparently random patterns of human life and death are increasingly viewed as predictable and calculable events. And once we have read our Max Weber, of course, all of this becomes understandable. For what we are witnessing here is nothing other than one further expression of that grand process which he referred to as 'rationalization'. A process which on the one hand is linked to the rational calculation of all possible outcomes of human action – or at least to the 'calculability of the most important technical factors' (Weber, 1930: 24) – and on the other to a deep-seated 'disenchantment of the world' (Weber, 1948: 155), in which there are no miracles, but merely calculable coincidences.

What is most interesting from our point of view, of course, is that this very same actuarial vision of life and death was also applied to other events – and especially those daily misfortunes which we term accidents. So the old Latin concept of *accidens* (which connoted chance, fortune, contingency, the unforeseen), was thereby dressed in a new garb of predicability and calculability. Contingency was stabilised.

ACCIDENTS

Those who remember *Double Indemnity* will recall the story line in which Mrs Dietrichson (Barbara Stanwyck) seeks to take out an accident policy on her husband. It is at that point that the insurance salesman, Walter Neff (played by Fred McMurray), almost intuitively realises that she is plotting something unpleasant – for accidents are rare events, and he knows that accidents on trains are even rarer (at least in Southern California *circa* 1943, if not on British Rail *circa* 1993). This notion that we can calculate with some precision the probabilities of accidents occurring in particular places and to particular groups of people is of course part of that rationalisation process of which I have just spoken. Indeed it represents a supreme example of Hacking's taming of chance, for it implies that we can somehow model unpredictability, the unforeseen, in some relatively accurate manner. For example, if we take the Poisson function.

$$\pi\ (\mathrm{x})\ =\ e^{-\mu}\ .\frac{n^x}{x!}$$

we should have a perfectly adequate model for predicting the rate at which random events (such as accidents) occur in any given population. The only unknown in the function is μ – which we can estimate from any empirical population distribution. To illustrate the point, I am going to discuss these, and associated problems, in relation to *General Household Survey* (GHS) data for 1987–9.[1]

In the 1987–9 GHS surveys, respondents were asked whether they had experienced any kind of accident in the three months prior to interview as a result of which they had sought medical treatment. Details concerning the nature of the sample and the questionnaire that was used are to be found in Breeze *et al.* (1991). The files on which this analysis is based (an 80 per cent sample of *ESRC Data Archive* files 2724 and 2679) contain the answers of some 51,080 individuals to this question and in those responses one can find recorded reference to 2,136 accidents. Using that information to form a maximum likelihood estimate for μ, we get 0.04181.

Table 11.1 Numbers of accidents reported by 51,080 respondents for a three-month period

Number of accidents per person	Reported	Predicted by Poisson model
0	48944	48988.044
1	2081	2048.521
≥ 2	55	43.435

Source: *ESRC Data Archive Files* for GHS 1987 and 1988–9 combined

Note: Chi-squared = 3.634 with 1 d.f. $0.1 < SP < 0.2$

The Poisson function then predicts the number of accidents for this population to be as indicated in Table 11.1. As we can see from the chi-square result, the model fits the data reasonably well. In fact this example serves to show how quite complex mathematical functions can be called upon to model so-called 'random' and rare events, and it is in that sense that we can speak of chance being tamed. Indeed so thorough has been the transformation in our understanding of chance that had this or some other probability distribution failed to fit the data we would have been inclined to argue that something other than 'chance' was involved in the distribution of accidents. That is to say, it is nowadays only when we cannot predict – only when we fail to find order and regularity – that we hold the hypothesis of a random distribution of events to be null and void. (This somewhat fascinating turn around in our comprehension of 'randomness' was in fact first remarked upon by Karl Pearson (1897, I: 11).) One need only add that it is usually possible to formulate far more complex models than the one above. And just to give the reader a taste of such possibilities I shall do little more than refer to a transport and road research report of 1991 wherein was included the following model – directed toward the frequency of road accidents:

$$Accident - 0.00633e^{(s+g)} (1 + 1.6pd)$$
$$(pb + 0.65pr + 0.88pm) M^{0.279}$$
$$\exp\left[\frac{b_1}{Ag} + \frac{b_2}{X + 2.6}\right]$$

Here, s and b_2 are variables related to gender; g and b_1 are related to socio-economic characteristics; pd is proportion of driving undertaken in the dark; pb, pr, pm refer to urban, rural, and motorway roads respectively; M is the distance driven annually in miles; Ag refers to driver's age; and X refers to years of driving experience (see Maycock *et al.* (1991) for a full explanation of the model).

Now, at the risk of scaring off those who are antithetical to a mathematical analysis of human affairs, I would in fact like to stay with my first example a little longer so as to highlight one or two further features of the mathematical process. The first concerns the fact that what we are looking at here is a *rate*. And a rate such as this is necessarily derived from the observation of collective processes – it is derived from a population. Indeed I have deliberately chosen the word 'collective' in accordance with a usage that was suggested by von Mises as far back as 1928. von Mises (1939) pointed out that a probability calculation involves the consideration of two sequences as follows:

(A)	0	1	1	0	1	0	0	0	0	1	0
(A')	0	1/2	2/3	1/2	3/5	1/2	3/7	3/8	1/3	2/5	4/11

At this stage we need to make note of a number of properties contained in these sequences. First of all we can see that the sequence labelled (A) is composed of nothing but zeros and ones. An empirical interpretation of such a sequence would be that an event (accident, death, birth) either occurs or does not occur, and in this particular sequence there is no apparent pattern – it looks random. The lower sequence labelled (A') is of course derived from the upper one. It tells us what proportion of ones occurs in the sequence to date. As we can see, (A') fluctuates – quite wildly. In the long run, however, we assume that the lower sequence will stabilize in some way – say at the probability of 0.5, 0.3, 0.04181 or whatever. And it is this long-run assessment that we refer to when we talk about the 'probability' of an event. In mathematical terms we might say that the probability coefficient represents the limit of relative frequency in a sequence. (Though this frequentist understanding is not the only way in which we can interpret the concept of probability.)

In terms of my example, of course, the final probability of 4/11 could have been derived from a number of different (A) sequences. For example, the upper sequence might have started off with four ones in a row, followed by seven zeros. Or four consecutive ones could have occurred in the middle of the list, and so on. The reason why I am labouring this point is simply in order to emphasise the fact that probability calculations refer to the collective and not to the individual occurrences. The sequence labelled (A) is, in that sense, undetermined, and even when the probability in a sequence has stabilised we cannot predict whether the next digit in the upper sequence will be a zero or a one. Indeed, in frequency theory 'probabilities cannot be ascribed to singular occurrences, but only to infinite sequences of occurrences or events' (Popper, 1959: 210).

When we apply these elementary mathematical lessons to an empirical population we can also see why it makes no sense to pin the probabilities derived from a collective sequence to a single person – whose future also remains indeterminate. Hence it cannot be used to predict which individuals will and will not have an accident. Indeed the probability of having an accident for any individual must either be 0 ('Dad. Look! No hands.') or 1 ('I told you not to do that you silly little bugger'). In this sense the accident rate rather like the death rate belongs to all of us, collectively. To apply probability calculations concerning death or accidents to specific individuals detached from the socially defined groups and sub-groups to which they belong – from what Popper (1959) once called the reference classes – would be thoroughly misleading. Misleading first in the sense that the probability calculations would suggest that there is something about the individuals (rather than the 'sequences' in terms of which they live) that would make them more or less prone to 'having an accident', and second because it would suggest that there is only one probability of the actual event taking place, (whereas, in fact, the same event can have different probabilities according to which particular reference class we are considering it in relation to). Naturally, the possibility exists that both the upper and the lower sequence eventually stabilise into a recognisable pattern, say 0, 1, 0, 1, 0, 1, 0, 1 ... 0, 1 – but it is difficult to think of any so-called health events that might look like this. (Though perhaps the patterns of birth of girls and boys come close to it.)

The second point that I wish to make in relation to my example is that the Poisson rate changes significantly for different sub-populations (reference classes) within the sample. As we can see from the information contained in Tables 11.2, 11.3 and 11.4, gender, age and occupational class, at least, seem to make a difference to the probabilities of 'having an accident'. This implies that there are significant deviations from the long-term average frequency in the mathematical series. In other words there are certain finite segments of the long chain of zeros and ones where the rate deviates from the average. Perhaps, for example, the overall Poisson process is made up of a series of 'mini' Poisson processes. And this in turn would suggest that the event space within which the process is operating has altered in someway. In other words chance may be at work, but it is only at work within the limits of certain parameters.

It seems likely, then, that what is happening here is that the environments in which the various sub-groups act out their lives are radically different – one from the other. (I use the term 'environment' in its widest possible sense to include elements of what anthropologists have called 'culture' – as well as visible material surroundings.) Thus males and females, young and old, manual and non-manual workers must be encountering different environments and thereby experiencing different accident rates. And what I wish to emphasise at this point is that the properties that enable us to predict things about the occurrence of accidents are all collective properties and not individual ones. That is, they involve features of collective, moral life – features whose presence is perhaps merely signalled through the age, sex and class variations.

All in all, then, we are thereby left with an apparent contradiction. On the one hand, accidents are things that happen to individuals, and on the other, they can only be predicted for populations – that is, as a rate. And they need to be understood (and in fact are understood by many professional groups) as a rate. To alter the rate, we would have somehow to alter the event space within which accidents occur.

Table 11.2 Proportions of male and female respondents reporting an accident during the three months before interview

Males	Females
0.0503	0.0339
(N = 24548)	(N = 26532)
z = 9.1792	p = 0.0000

Source: GHS files for 1987 and 1988–9 combined

Table 11.3 Proportions of manual (Social Class I, II, IIIM) and non-manual (Social Class IIINM, IV, V) respondents reporting an accident during the three months before interview

Manual	Non-manual
0.0468	0.0349
(N = 29877)	(N = 21203)
z = 6.6232	p = 0.0000

Source: GHS files for 1987 and 1988–9 combined

Table 11.4 Proportions of respondents reporting an accident during the three months before interview by age group

Age	p	N	95% confidence interval
0–24	0.0561	17514	(0.0527, 0.0595)
25–49	0.0403	17383	(0.0374, 0.0432)
50–74	0.0258	12923	(0.0231, 0.0285)
75+	0.0371	3260	(0.0306, 0.0436)

Source: GHS files for 1987 and 1988–9 combined

HEALTH PROMOTION AND ACCIDENTS

'In theory at least, all accidents are preventable.'

(Department of Health, 1992a)

This statement epitomises the modernist project. For to prevent all accidents, one would in practice have to control the environment absolutely and in every detail. The fact that the Department of Health considers such an outcome to be possible 'in theory' is of course interesting in itself. It is not, however, a possibility on which I wish to dwell in this paper. Instead I prefer to take up two other observations relating to the *Health of the Nation* document. The first relates to what we might call (following Bauman (1992b)) the 'deconstruction' of contingency. The second involves the imputation of causes.

In his *Mortality, Immortality and Other Life Strategies*, Bauman (1992b) talks about the deconstruction of death. By that he means the process whereby the massive, insurmountable problem of human mortality has been reduced to myriad lesser (health) problems – all of which are 'in theory' conquerable. For example, if we take the WHO categories of causes of death, injury and diseases we have some 999.999 possible causes. Since nearly all of these causes refer to disease entities – no one can die of old age, for example – and since we 'know' that science can (in theory) conquer all, modern cultures have developed and even encouraged a tendency in their members to believe that death itself is conquerable. Therein lies Bauman's process of deconstruction.

We can extend Bauman's ideas a little further and suggest that by incorporating accidents under the heading of 'health problem', modern societies seek to deconstruct contingency. That is, we are encouraged to believe that all forms of fate, chance and misfortune can 'in theory' be controlled or modified through the alteration of personal health behaviours so that nothing uncontrollable need ever occur in a single human life as long as we 'behave properly'. In that sense the statement that opens this sub-section can be more properly seen as a component of a modernist cosmology rather than as a serious comment on the nature of empirical reality.

The second implication of *The Health of the Nation... And You* (Department of Health, 1992b) involves the question of causation. For the document includes at least two 'targets'. The first calls for a reduction in the rates of accidental death among children and elderly people by at least one third. The second demands a reduction of rates of accidental death among young people by at least one quarter. (Note the emphasis on *rates* here.) Since 'very few accidents are due solely to chance' (Department of Health, 1992a: 10), the implication is that these targets can be achieved by means of planned human intervention in the respective causal chains. It is, I think, in the analysis of the presumed causes that further essential features of modernist and postmodernist cosmology appear.

'Cause and effect: such a duality probably never exists.' Thus spake Nietzsche in *The Gay Science* (1974: 112) – though real live human beings, of course, seem to be incapable of thinking in any other terms. What is of interest, however, lies not so much in the fact that human beings think in terms of causation, but in the structure and content of their specific explanations (Green, this volume). In this respect we can see reflected in *The Health of the Nation... And You*, a historically peculiar form of causal logic. For example, the document urges its readers to 'fit a smoke detector', 'beware of the chip pan', 'beware of damaged carpets', 'make sure that there is good lighting in hall ways and stairs', and so on. In other words it seeks to reduce the numbers of accidents by correcting numerous technical shortcomings that are to be found in individual households. For it is presumably in such contexts that the causes of accidents are to be found.

Now it is not for any sociologist to suggest that such a line of reasoning is in some way in error, but it is incumbent on sociology perhaps to highlight the limitations of such ways of thinking. For what is happening here is that the causal contributions of what we have previously referred to as 'the environment' are being eclipsed by the analysis of mere technical considerations. More specifically, (and recalling the claims concerning the social distribution of accidents above), we can further see that questions relating to such things as the unequal distribution of safe environments or the unequal distribution of resources in general (new cars, forms of heating fuel, kitchen technology and so on) are entirely ignored. Yet – on the basis both of the mathematics and of common sense moral discourse – we would have as much right to argue that it was factors in the wider environment that truly caused accidents as it was the chip pan, the hall light, the ragged carpet or whatever.

As I have already stated above, this is not to suggest that the forms of sociological explanation hinted at herein are in any sense superior to those contained in the Department of Health booklet. Indeed in both cases the eschewing of final causes as possible explanations of accidents betrays the modern origins of both kinds of argument. But it is I think clear that the substitution of relatively simple questions concerning technical procedures (mainly in the home) for bigger and broader considerations of moral discourse expresses very clearly a universal characteristic of modernist and perhaps postmodernist thinking – namely a predilection to concentrate only upon that which can be easily controlled. In so doing, such forms of thought reduce various kinds of collective moral (political) problems to mere questions of technical rationality. So in that sense problems are posed in terms of a privatised morality and the technical (in)competence of individuals, rather than in terms of collective considerations. (This tendency was even more marked in *Prevention and Health: Everybody's Business* (DHSS, 1976a).)

This latter point is, perhaps, best understood in relation to my final, and somewhat stark example. It concerns the reported death rate from road accidents in Northern Ireland 1968–91. (My opening date is deliberately selected to coincide with the commencement of 'the troubles'.) We can see at once from Figure 11.1 a very sharp rise in such deaths during the early 1970s and a series of smaller fluctuations thereafter. More interestingly, we see an echo of this pattern just below it in the death rate from homicides – almost as if the reverberations from the lower pattern were prompting the rhythm of the upper one. In fact, the correlation coefficient between the two sets of figures was calculated as being 0.663. I am not, however, truly interested in exploring the relationships between the two patterns exhibited in Figure 11.1, though I am certain that one could interpret them both as being the product of a common cause – namely, of what happens in a society when, to quote the inimitable verse of W.B. Yeats (1973 [1920])

Things fall apart; the centre cannot hold;
Mere anarchy is loosed upon the world,
The blood-dimmed tide is loosed, and everywhere
The ceremony of innocence is drowned.

Instead I focus on what would and what would not constitute a plausible source of explanations for each trend. Starting with the homicide rate I would like to suggest that if I sought to explain the variations in that rate according to personal failings – failure to fit a bomb alarm, failing to belt up one's flak jacket, or injudicious use of timing devices – I would very properly be laughed out of court. For it is certain that whatever exact form an acceptable explanation of such events were to take, it would at the very least make some mention of the wider political and cultural factors that gave rise to the massive increase in homicides that is evident in the graph. Somewhat surprisingly, however, when we read explanatory accounts of the upper graph – as may, for example be found in the Annual (RUC) Report of Road Traffic Accident Statistics – we find no mention of politics or culture in any sense whatsoever. Instead we see the trends attributed to technical changes in the law, or policing arrangements, or the personal behaviour of motorists. Whilst I would not for one minute dispute the role of drink driving laws, the fitting of car seat belts and attention to speed limits as important factors in any consideration of road accident rates, I would dispute the application of double standards to apparently interlinked trends. In short, if a satisfactory explanation of the trends in the homicide rate calls for reference to what I have previously termed collective social factors – then so too would a satisfactory explanation of trends in the road accident (death) rate.

To sum up then, we might say that the authors of *The Health of the Nation* have chosen to discuss (and thereby explain) accidents in terms of an individualistic and technical framework – forsaking all reference to the nature of the collective activities that impinge on accidental events. In so doing, they have not only given a full-blooded expression to modernist culture, but they have also substituted a consideration of a limited and personal environment (because, as we all know, accidents occur 'in the home', 'on the road', 'at work') for a consideration of collective, structural factors which are equally deserving of serious consideration in the explanatory framework.

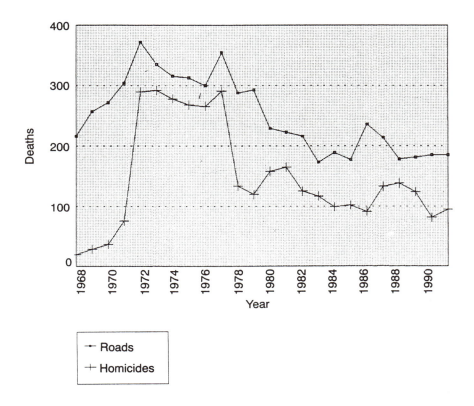

Figure 11.1 Deaths from road accidents and homicides in Northern Ireland 1968–91
Source: Annual Reports of the Registrar General (DHSS, 1992) and the Royal Ulster Constabulary (1992)

CONCLUSION

Our entire concept of an accident rate is a product of modernist discourse. It is an expression of that rationalisation process in terms of which all forms of magic, fate, luck and chance have been rendered irrelevant – a process that Weber considered as one of the roots of that 'disillusioned and pessimistically inclined individualism' (Weber, 1930: 105) which characterises the modern world. One might say that the growth of the insurance industry is in many ways the firmest organisational expression of this rationalisation process.

Yet, whilst modernism has generated an image of a determinate and controllable universe, postmodernism has rendered the understanding of the world in terms of *collective* social properties improper. The postmodernist world is, when all is said and done, composed only of isolated consumers. Consequently, perhaps, postmodernist ideology has turned a collective problem of moral dimensions (namely a problem involving such things as social cohesion, access to safe environments, and plentiful resources) into a personal problem of technical failings. *The Health of the Nation . . . And You* is in that sense as much a postmodernist as a modernist handbook.

NOTES

1 Material from the GHS made available through the Office of Population Censuses and Surveys and the ESRC Data Archive has been used by permission of the Controller of H.M. Stationery Office. The interpretation of the material, however, remains the sole responsibility of the author.

Chapter 12

London dentist in HIV scare
HIV and dentistry in popular discourse

Nicki Thorogood

INTRODUCTION

On Friday 12 March 1993 the *Evening Standard* publicity boards proclaimed 'London Dentist in HIV Scare'. The newspaper's headline ran 'I worked on despite HIV says dentist'. This was during a week in which there had been publicity about the death of a GP from AIDS and the disclosure that a consultant gynaecologist was seriously ill with an AIDS-related disorder. It was followed in the Sunday papers by reports that the death of another hospital doctor had recently come to light.

These 'human interest' stories are contextualised with the 'expert rulings' (General Dental Council, 1989; Department of Health, 1993b) on disclosure and on safety procedures regarding health workers. Given that the only known case of patients/clients becoming infected as a result of treatment is that of the US dentist David Acer, we wondered just what popular views were about HIV and dental treatment.

As a consequence, the UMDS Unit of Dental Public Health undertook a survey of 102 people 'in the street'. This took place on two dates in May 1993 (6 and 19) largely due to organisational demands. Whilst media coverage on HIV in general sustained a high profile during this period, there was a slight lull in the coverage of HIV and health care workers as an issue. A possible effect of this timing was that the issue was not at the forefront of people's minds and the media coverage was not providing them with ready rhetoric or received wisdom in their answers. It did, however, mean it was a recent enough issue for most people to feel they could give informed answers.

METHOD

The survey was carried out in two distinct geographical areas – Dartford and Tunbridge Wells, which differ in their estimated level of health demand and in their mix of population. People were selected on an *ad hoc* basis and in total 102 people were questioned, 51 at each site. Most people (70 per cent) had visited the dentist in the last year. We used a short questionnaire with an introductory section asking for gender, age, occupation, postcode (to exclude non-local residents) and we also asked about frequency of attendance at the dentist. We then asked nine further questions concerning HIV and dentistry. Statistically, there was no significant difference for any of the questions when analysed by gender, site or attendance, although age did show some significance. Over half of the people interviewed thought a General Dental Practitioner (GDP) should be allowed to go on working and (fore)saw very little difficulty in dentists being forced to disclose their HIV status, nor reciprocally, in disclosures of their own status. Indeed most people said they would be prepared to be treated by a GDP known or suspected to be HIV+. However, the data drawn on here is largely that given as 'supporting remarks', those throwaway comments made by people in the course of their 'real' interview as part of the street survey.[1]

A THEORETICAL FRAMEWORK

The quantitative results indicate a fairly rational, liberal attitude which is perhaps in contrast to our expectations of the 'popular discourse' of the general public. These opinions are apparently derived from a discourse that presumes a fair and rational world in which decisions are made and actions are taken in the light of full knowledge and calculable risks. This seems somewhat at odds with the kind of hysterical 'tabloid' (and often 'broadsheet' as well) response that characterises press reports and which is taken for granted as the 'lay' view.

Does this then mean that we ('the expert commentators'; 'we' who know best what the 'real' risks are; 'we' who experience daily the consequences of oppression) should not despair? That 'things' (that is, public opinion, prejudice, homophobia, irrationality and so on) are not as bad as we had thought; that the 'lay' view is more informed, more considered, better educated (ah! so our campaigns have been successful), more rational than we had dared to hope? Maybe. Maybe not. More likely, is that many of the responses are the 'public account' (Cornwell, 1984) that broadly reflects the 'socially acceptable' viewpoint and the desire not to appear overly ignorant.

What seems to me to be really interesting about the responses to the survey are not the answers to the formal questions but the 'supporting remarks', the qualifications of responses and the clarifications. These seem to me to belie a different order. Is this simply a slip into the quest for 'authenticity', the underlying 'true' meaning? I hope not. I hope it is merely articulating aspects of a hidden discourse, an oppositional framework, rendered invisible in the survey setting – but not 'hidden' in the private setting of, say, conversations with those who acknowledge some shared values (maybe workmates, teammates (generally men), friends, neighbours or family members (women)). Or in those startling conversational remarks made by 'service providers' to clients. It is this arena of 'common sense' views that the (tabloid) press tap into and which constructs and confirms categories of 'normal' and 'deviant'.[2]

There are, I think, at least two layers to the cake (discourse) here (as everywhere); there are, as I have suggested, the 'public' and the 'private' aspects. In the responses that we have considered so far the public account, situated in a discourse of rationality, is to the fore. This is an entirely expected aspect of 'modernity' (Weber, 1963; Rotter, 1982; Giddens, 1991; Green, 1992b) whether it is seen as an aspect of 'progress' with the possibility of either positive or negative consequences, or whether it is theorised as a social construction. As Green (1992b) notes, our modern belief system has not universally been held to be rational but whether or not one accepts rationality as the truth (or the 'scientific'), few would contest its place as the dominant discourse of Western thought.

To fracture this understanding, to take 'rational discourse' as only one discourse (albeit the most public, the most legitimate) allows the space for the theoretical consideration of the private account, the irrational (or anti-rational?) discourse, rather than simply consigning it to the irrelevant; an anachronistic hangover from a prerational thought system. To problematise 'rationality' may give us a way into understanding the private accounts also given in this survey.

I am particularly interested in the operation of 'anti-rational' discourse in informing 'individual behaviour' and decision making; it seems to me to be largely ignored but very pertinent to public health and health promotion. This chapter is an attempt to theorise the place of 'trust', 'fate' and 'risk' in personal decision making about about 'health'. As Giddens, discussing 'fate' remarks:

> To live in the universe of high modernity is to live in an environment of chance and risk, the inevitable concomitants of a system geared to the domination of nature and the reflexive making of history. Fate and destiny have no formal part to play in such a system, which operates (as a matter of principle) via what I shall call open human control of the natural and social worlds. The universe of future events is open to be shaped by human intervention – with limits which, as far as possible, are regulated by risk assessment. Yet the notions of fate and destiny have by no means disappeared in modern societies, and an investigation into their nature is rich with implications for the analysis of modernity and self-identity.
>
> (Giddens 1991: 107)

The calculation of one's personal as opposed to statistical safety is, it seems, the key tension between the two discourses. It is apparent in those daily risks we take – when driving or crossing the road, when eating 'unhealthy' food, giving children sweets, smoking a cigarette: just *one* won't matter; my grandfather smoked all his life and lived to 90; you've got to die of something . . . Indeed it hinges on that old anthropological debate of explaining why me, and why now? Or in this case why *should* it be me and why *should* it be this time that this one relatively safe act becomes the dangerous one? It is these considerations that I have called here 'anti-rational discourses'. These 'alternative' discourses, I suggest, are the central tension for the project of 'public health' (public/private; rational/anti-rational) because they lie outside the rational epidemiological arena and draw upon other discourses to assess and legitimise it. Giddens sums this up: 'Information derived from abstract systems may help in risk assessment but it is the individual concerned who has to run the risks in question' (Giddens, 1991: 114).

The presence of alternative discourses (whether we call them 'anti-rational' or not) in popular culture implicitly compromises rationality's claims. It suggests that, as Green remarks, rationality (as embodied by Western science) is not inevitably all-conquering, but is inherently precarious and liable to chaos (Green, 1994).

So the theoretical framework I am suggesting here is that the survey questions were, for the most part, answered from within the rational 'public' discourse but that the supplementary remarks tended to articulate private accounts located in other discourses such as fate, risk, trust and morality.

ANTI-RATIONAL DISCOURSES

A preliminary analysis of these glimpses into the 'private' accounts cannot elicit more than an indication of what might constitute these alternative discourses; however, a number of themes are revealed. There is a predominance of remarks that refer to 'taking the proper precautions' and to being 'clean'. These were generally made to support the view that a dentist should not be obliged to disclose (and were therefore volunteered by the interviewee before being asked during the course of the interview):

'Not if gloves are worn.'
'It should be quite safe in the practice.'
'All dentists should be tested and checked they are using precautions.'
'I saw a programme on TV and if they wear protection there is no harm to me.'

Such qualifiers were also made when discussing whether or not GDPs should be barred from practice if they are HIV+, and when discussing the prospect of treatment by a dentist known to be HIV+:

'With proper precautions.'
'As long as they are using protection.'
'Assuming they take precautions.'
'They should provide extra precautions.'

This, I suggest, picks up on rationality – it would be unreasonable to say no (although calculably safer) and it would appear dangerously ill-informed not to qualify their liberal perspective. But there is the quality of a ritualised but specifically meaningless phrase here, like 'have a nice day' or 'see you soon'. 'Protection' and 'precautions' come from the language of sexual risk-taking (these comments do tend to conjure up the image of a male dentist using a condom rather than the generalised use of latex gloves).

Also apparent from these comments is the perception that 'precautions' are taken to protect the patient instead of the more likely case that 'precautions' protect the dentist. 'Precautions' essentially covers the respondent against appearing too ignorant or from having to confront the issue (for example having to ask their dentist about cross infection procedures). Indeed, 94 per cent of the sample recalled their dentist wearing gloves at their last visit. Also in this form of assessment of relative risk or safety were comments about hygiene, sterility and cleanliness. While this too relates to rational discourse on cross infection it also recalls Mary Douglas (1984) in *Purity and Danger*, for example:

'I assumed everything was clean.'
'He wears gloves, uses a mask and a sterilising unit, all you would expect from a *good* dentist.' (Emphasis added)
'He is very clean.'
'It is so clean even the paintwork is spotless.'
'He is a particularly nice dentist, everything is covered up.'

The 'precautions' taken become elided with one's sense of the goodness or cleanliness of the dentist him- or herself. But it was clearly a hard decision for those who made qualifying remarks; there was a strong intimation of the attempt to weigh up what you know to be true (rationality) and what you feel:

'No [they shouldn't be prevented from practising], although I would be nervous.'

and

'I would like to say "yes" but it has to be "no".'

and, perhaps exemplifying the private accounts

'No way' [would the respondent have treatment from an HIV+ dentist].

So, in terms of calculating patients' own risk from the dentist, I suggest that 'taking precautions' appeals to both discourses. On the one hand it alludes to a knowable, calculable and therefore predictable risk of cross infection against which suitable 'precautions' can be taken, thereby minimising the danger. This is the rational model identified by Giddens (1991) as characterising 'modernity'. However, alongside this I suggest 'taking precautions' acts to distance the decision making; to shift the responsibility for risk-taking (and risk assessment) to the dentist. It makes the patients' problem go away and suggests a much more fatalistic outlook:

'What you don't know you don't worry about.'
'I tend not to worry – you would worry over everything otherwise.'

This too, according to Giddens, is a consequence of the rational discourse. He suggests that: 'Fatalism is the refusal of modernity – a repudiation of a controlling origination to the future in favour of an attitude which lets events come as they will' (Giddens, 1991: 110).

Thus in the comments made in responses to other questions we find the discourse of 'trust' emerging in the comments which appeal to (i) the 'good' dentist and (ii) the location of moral obligation and professional responsibility with the dentist and lay responsibilities and rights with the patient.

A GOOD DENTIST

A 'good dentist' was one that you knew.

'It depends how long I had known the dentist.'
'Yes because if he was a good dentist he would be very careful anyway.'
'If it was my dentist, yes, but not a new one.'
'Yes if it was my own dentist that I knew.'
'Yes if I had known him for a while.'
'It depends on how well I knew the dentist.'
'As long as he was my own dentist.'

This recalls the findings of the Women, Risk and AIDS Project (WRAP) (Holland et al., 1990), where it was found that young women's commitment to safer sex decreases with the length of a relationship. Relaxing 'precautions' was an indication of trust/'love' and an unwillingness to take risks reflected badly on young women ('if you really loved/trusted me you would'). As has been noted by both Balint (1957) and Cornwell (1984), a 'good' doctor is one you have known for a long time.

The concept of trust that is invoked here is, I think, drawn from an anti-rational discourse; it appeals to finer feelings and moral responsibility. You do not know, in the sense of calculable risk, but you know in the sense of making moral judgements.

Smithson's (1985) development of a social theory of ignorance starts to theorise how expert knowledge implies 'trust' on the part of those who are socially constructed as ignorant. It is a key feature of the lay/professional relationship. You do not know, in the sense of possessing expert knowledge, whether your car engine does need what the garage mechanic says, or the plumber, etc. (Smithson, 1985: 163). You consult a doctor or a dentist for their expert opinion and you have to believe that they are acting in your best interests. This is largely a matter of trust based on sets of implicit rules. To quote the *Daily Telegraph* on 11 March 1993 in an editorial piece entitled 'HIV and a question of trust':

> The onus is also on every medical professional in a high-risk group to arrange to be tested regularly but voluntarily. Although it is clear not all of them are doing so. The public is obliged to place extraordinary trust in the medical professions. The professions in their turn must go to extraordinary lengths to ensure that this trust is deserved.

So a patient has to place trust in a dentist. But how is this to be gauged except through 'evidence' which appeals to the intuitive but which is couched in the rational language of 'cleanliness and hygiene'. Or from evidence drawn from experience: 'I've known him a long time.' As the quote expresses it, it is a dependent relationship; we must place our trust in the dentist but the dentist must demonstrate her or his trustworthiness.

This trustworthiness is apparently a consequence of 'professional responsibility', and many of the comments refer to this:

> 'It should be the dentist's duty to the patient.'
> 'It would be their responsibility to tell me.'
> 'Yes he should be responsible enough to take the necessary precautions.'
> 'Yes if he was conscientious in cross infection control.'
> 'Yes if he was approved by the BDC.'

And again this notion seems to indicate that the patient's safety is beyond his or her control – that the risk can be better assessed by the dentist/professional and that there is a moral obligation on the part of the dentist to minimise the risk to the respondent personally. So this is an appeal to the professional ethos. Is this rational or not? This also occurs in comments regarding disclosure:

> 'I would expect them to be responsible enough to tell the patient.'
> 'It should be the dentist's duty to the patient.'
> 'If you had a good dentist I feel certain he would tell you.'
> 'He has a duty and a responsibility.'
> 'Mixed feelings, everyone has a right to know but I would never think to ask my own dentist.'

'I hope he would take all the right precautions – they are just as much at risk as us.'

It is evident that this trust has been betrayed from the quote from Sherry Johnson (Acer's sixth 'victim'): 'He may have done it deliberately we heard but we had faith in what the medical establishment was telling us. We didn't panic' (*Mail on Sunday*, 25 May 1993). Again this suggests that the patient's safety is beyond her control – that risk can be better assessed by the professional dentist and that there is a moral obligation on the part of the dentist to minimise the risk to the respondent personally.

THE MORAL PATIENT

The notion of rights was most in evidence in the responses to the questions of whether patients' HIV status should be routinely checked:

'Yes they have a right to know.'
'Yes he has a right to ask you and you have a right to ask him.'
'Fair's fair, if we want to know if they are then they should know if we are.'

Regarding patients' disclosure it came out strongly that it would be the right thing to do:

'It's only fair.'
'It's the right thing to do.'
'I'd have a moral obligation to myself.'
'It's not something to hide.'
'I would worry about passing it on/putting others at risk.'

Disclosure (both ways) acts to make the risk more calculable. Maybe it also depends on beliefs about 'rights' and 'duties' as a way of assessing those of whom you have no personal knowledge (for example, other dentists and patients) and therefore cannot trust. If you cannot place trust in them then you have to trust that the discourse of 'rights and duties' will ensure a sense of moral/professional responsibility in them to make your risk as 'knowable' as possible. (So then you too have to say you will operate by that code and therefore have to disclose or say you will – fair's fair.)

One theme running through the press cuttings was that of 'secrecy': moral outrage at any element of 'secrecy' which could possibly be constructed or discerned (again, see Smithson (1985) for an explication of privacy and secrecy as techniques of control). Secrecy is an anathema to 'trust' and again this is couched in terms of 'rights' and 'responsibilities'. This is illustrated by the following extract from an article in *Gay Scotland* quoted by Esteban (1993): 'Later, the paper revealed that the doctor had been: "convicted of importuning 30 years ago". The Sun, no doubt, would argue that the public has a *right to know* such details of a man who is now dying in hospital', and: 'The man himself comes across as being a *responsible* human being, whose only concern is his patients' (Esteban, 1993: 22).

The estimates of risk in the encounter are instructive. People have some notion of the global scale being low and therefore risk being small (although the actual figures they suggest translate quite large). This is perhaps reflected by their assessment of their own safety as generally safe. Their specific judgement of their own safety is derived less from the global picture and more from what they know about their own dental encounters. But then comes the crunch: you 'know' all you can; how then do you decide what personally to do? This, suggests Giddens, is the place of 'fate' as an alternative anti-rational discourse. Information derived from abstract systems may help in risk assessment, but it is the individual concerned who has to run the risks in question (Giddens, 1991: 114).

As the *Sun* editorial (31 May 1993) challenged: if experts tell us the risk is negligible, then, 'Every health chief should carry a card welcoming treatment by an AIDS infected doctor.' This encapsulates the tension between calculable risk and personal fate, the small statistical risk and the potentially enormous personal consequence. Sherry Johnson (*Mail on Sunday*, 25 May 1993) brings this home with force when she comments on the fact that only half of Acer's 2,000 patients have been tested for HIV: 'statistically that means there are probably six more walking around carrying his virus'.

Perhaps what we can conclude from this is that trust and responsibility are the flip side of risk; they are the means of managing the modern problem of consistently evaluating risks:

> Within the settings of daily life, basic trust is expressed as a bracketing-out of possible events or issues which could, in certain circumstances, be cause for alarm ... The 'uneventful' character of much of day-to-day life is the result of a skilled watchfulness that only long schooling produces [*Umwelt*], and is crucial to the protective cocoon which all regularised action presumes ... The protective cocoon is the mantle of trust that makes possible the sustaining of a viable *Umwelt*.
>
> (Giddens, 1991: 127–9)

CONCLUSION

A central tenet of 'modernity' is rationality and that demands the calculation of risk. HIV presents a dilemma in that it is an incalculable risk (on an individual level – unlike, for instance, 'getting pregnant') and that the personal consequences are high. This makes appeals to rationality meaningless and decision making is based on 'feeling' located in other, anti-rational discourses such as trust and morality. This might go some way towards explaining the survey results in that answering abstract questions can be done rationally and therefore appear quite 'liberal' but assessing personal risk and danger is another matter. Popular discourse around HIV and dentistry is a shining example of the fragility of rationality and of the coexistence of contemporary anti-rational alternative discourses. It is these which we see underpinning (most) media coverage.

NOTES

1 The following gives a quantitative indication of the sorts of responses made to the questions. The data are not statistically representative, but are provided here in summary for information and in order to contextualise the qualitative comments of the respondents upon which the rest of the chapter draws.

Should a dentist be obliged (forced) to tell their patients that they are HIV+?: Overall most people (80.4 per cent) thought a dentist should be obliged (forced) to disclose his or her own HIV status. Most people also thought that a dentist should be allowed to continue working, albeit with some restrictions (50 per cent said 'yes', 15.7 per cent said 'it depends' and 34.3 per cent said 'no'). However, it was the younger age group who were most likely to make the qualifying remarks such as: 'If they are wearing gloves and protecting the patient there is no need (to disclose their own status)'.

Should dentists check patients' HIV status?: Regarding patients' HIV status, most people (66.3 per cent) thought a dentist should check all patients, a further 5.9 per cent thought 'certain types' should be checked and 27.7 per cent thought a dentist should not check. Significantly, 22.3 per cent of these were in the younger age group. Possibly related to this finding is that whilst most people also said they would tell their dentist if they were HIV+ (76.2 per cent) and the numbers in each age group were similar, of the remaining 23 people who would not disclose their positive status, 22 were in the younger age group. This leads to the speculation that younger people have given the issue of their own HIV status more serious thought and their answers reflect the higher degree to which they feel themselves to be at risk.

Would you be prepared to be treated by a dentist who you knew to be HIV+?: People were divided fairly evenly by gender, age, site and attendance as to whether they would be prepared to be treated by a dentist known to be HIV+, although this was qualified by 11.8 per cent of the sample.

If you suspected your dentist might be HIV+ would you still be prepared to have treatment?: The decision was apparently less clear if you only suspected the possibility of your dentist being HIV+. Still, many (47.5 per cent) said they would be prepared but of these 66 per cent were in the younger age group, whereas, of the 36.4 per cent who would not, 61 per cent were in the older age group. The remaining 15.2 per cent of the sample qualified their decision.

What precautions does your dentist take to avoid passing infections from one patient to another?: In line with the findings of Humphris *et al.* (1993) most people said they recalled their dentist taking precautions (for example, 94 per cent said their dentist wore gloves at their last visit), one person had witnessed cling film being used and two people had seen the dentist cleaning the chair. However, Humphris *et al.* (1993) suggest that this is more related to the desire of the respondents to believe that precautions are being taken, or to give the 'right answer' than the veracity of the statement. A further 67 per cent of our sample mentioned other precautions that were taken. These were mostly the wearing of a mask and/or sterilising equipment or the use of obviously sterile equipment (for example, needles in unopened packets).

How safe do you feel when visiting the dentist that the dentist has taken precautions against passing any infection on to you?: There were no significant differences in any respect with levels of perceived safety amongst the sample group. Indeed, 57 per cent of people felt very safe, 40 per cent quite safe, 3 per cent quite unsafe and none very unsafe.

2 I was shocked and depressed to see the press cuttings related to HIV when researching this paper – two D-ring binder files of A4 paper collected since March 1993. Shocked at the volume and depressed at the salacious, sordid, homophobic and pejorative nature of the articles. I had not previously realised the extent to which HIV/AIDS and anti-lesbian and gay utterances were needed/produced/used as a tool through which to construct and reconstruct the 'normal' world. I simply had not realised it was that important. Perhaps this too underscores the fragility of the dominant rational discourse.

Part IV

Health promotion, consumption and lifestyle

Chapter 13

In the name of health[1]

Barry Glassner

INTRODUCTION

For better or worse, we Americans have become obsessed with our bodies.

Some say such an obsession is clearly for the better. Health promoters point out that we are exercising more, keeping our weight down, and eating more wholesome meals. But critics say the current emphasis on the body is turning us into shallow, addicted narcissists who care about nothing beyond our own gratifications.

I say both views are based on the same faulty assumption: that an interest in the body is entirely a self-centred act.

It is for profoundly *social* reasons that we have directed so much attention to our bodies in the 1970s and 1980s. The body boom may *look* individualist, but in this case looks are deceiving. To be sure, the decision to have cosmetic surgery or to lift weights is made by an individual, and some of the pathologies of the age, such as exercise addiction and anorexia, are borne by individuals. But changes in society are very much implicated. As women's roles shifted, eating disorders became more common; as America sought to regain its might after the Vietnam War, the musclebound look grew popular.

What is more, when individuals set out to improve their bodies, usually they opt for social, not solitary, means. They enrol in health clubs or weight-loss programmes. Or they develop relationships with professionals – exercise instructors, diet doctors, cosmetic surgeons.

And people decide to alter their appearance not at indiscriminate points in their lives but most commonly when their social circumstances are changing.

'Women come to me at pivotal moments,' said Allison, a beauty-make-over specialist I interviewed in New York. 'Probably half of my clients are going through divorces. They're ready to give off a whole new set of signals, but they need a little help making it work. They're getting into circulation again and have visions of becoming glamorous and sexy. Or they're going more into their careers and need a bolder look.'

Other clients of Allison's seek revision rather than metamorphosis. 'A lot of women,' she reported, 'will say, "I got married and I had a kid and I dropped out for a while, but now my son's a toddler and I'm getting a part-time job and I want to update my image." Or sometimes college students will come to me when they're about to graduate, to professionalise their style before they go into the job market.'

She has also worked with women who use her services as a *stimulus* to change: 'They feel stuck. They look in the mirror and they feel ugly. They hate their bodies and they hate their clothes. They may love their babies and their husbands, but they're fighting with them too, because they feel taken for granted. They want to do something to effect a change, so they come to me to make them feel better.

'Once they look better they act like different people. They get along better with their kids, and their husbands start noticing them again.'

Some people alter their appearance to test whether they are capable of new challenges. 'A lot of times the makeover is a springboard that leads to other accomplishments,' said Allison. 'They figure if they had the nerve to go through with the makeover, they can go out and get a new job too . . . or dump the man who's been mistreating them. They get positive feedback from others, and it gives them the nerve to do other things.'

Cosmetic surgeons give similar reports. According to a study from Harvard Medical School (Belfer *et al.*, 1979), a substantial percentage of patients choose to have cosmetic surgery for reasons they are unable to face at the time but which reveal themselves later. Soon after the operation, they make a major life change, such as filing for divorce.

MORE THAN A HAIRCUT

Some body remakers are acutely aware that they provide social services to their clients. An electrologist named Karen, whom I interviewed at her office in Greenwich Village, sees many of her clients regularly for months on end, and frequently finds herself playing social worker on their behalf.

'For example,' Karen explained, 'one of my clients will tell me she and her husband are moving to the suburbs. Then another will come along who's just gotten divorced and needs a smaller place to live. So – to protect the confidentiality of my clients – I'll tell the second woman that I was at the health club yesterday and somebody was talking about giving up her apartment at such-and-such a location.

'Or somebody will be bitching that her younger brother the accountant never gets any dates. I'll give her the phone number of one of my clients – and I have *loads* in this category – who is a single woman looking for a stable man. To be discreet, I'll say she's in my aerobics dance class.'

Karen described her clients as women on the make in the business or theatre worlds, who go to her (and to cosmetic surgeons, personal trainers and weight reducers) because they don't want anything unsightly to stand between them and a six-figure-a-year income. But they get much more for their $35 per half-hour than just an electrocution of their hair follicles. In addition to her networking service, Karen listens appreciatively as they relate their most personal psychological, marital and financial problems. She has heard everything from minute-by-minute accounts of secret sexual rendezvous to the intimate details of insider stock trades.

It is common knowledge that electrologists, hairdressers, manicurists and masseuses function in our culture as surrogate psychiatrists and trusted friends. The usual explanation is that a majority of the population either cannot afford or does not know how to locate appropriate confidants. In many marriages and friendships, unspoken rules prohibit 'heavy' talk; and with work colleagues the dangers of revealing oneself may be great.

The body remakers I have interviewed, including Karen, give a second reason why people tell all to their hairdressers. They say that a person feels a kind of intimacy toward someone who has been allowed access to his or her body. After all, the body is the most private and personal of possessions; once you've turned *that* over to a stranger, the unloading of a few skeletons from your closet is no big deal.

I think there is a still less conscious reason as well. On some level, we envision these people as having special powers. Rationally, we know they can do no more than sharpen our appearance, but *ir*rationally we believe they can change our lives. We imagine them capable of making us into – in the words of an advertisement for a cosmetic surgery centre in Minneapolis – 'some body new'. Obviously (so reasons our subconscious), anyone who can transform us from one type of person into another must be able to readjust us emotionally as part of the package.

Karen, unlike the vast majority of body remakers, actually has some training in counselling. She was a psychiatric social worker, serving as a nurse at an inner-city psychiatric hospital. She had spent half a dozen years in the place, was on the verge of turning 30, and felt herself slowly simmering into a fully fledged burnout. Most of the patients, poor and suffering from schizophrenia, had been through the system many times. The best a staffer could hope for was to make it through a whole week without violence.

One day in 1981 a well-dressed but terribly agitated woman was admitted to the facility. 'Give me a razor! Give me a razor!' she shouted over and over. Karen ignored her at first, but when she did not let up after an hour, she went in to talk to her. 'She was sitting on the edge of the bed,' Karen remembered, 'and I noticed she had a whole chin full of hair. She had obviously been in a psychotic state for a week or so and had stopped taking care of herself. By the time she got to the hospital she was starting to come out of her psychosis, and she must have caught a glimpse of her face in a mirror.

'I was ahead on my paperwork for the day, so I just went to the supply cabinet, got a safety razor, took her to the bathroom, and shaved her chin.

'The minute the hair was off, she was a different person. She relaxed, she spoke coherently. My supervisor gave me hell about it, said that I'd taken a terrible risk, but it was probably the most effective therapy that woman had had in years.'

Hair removal will not often bring a highly disturbed patient back to earth. But more than a few progressive psychiatric hospitals employ full-time cosmetologists. After all, an important step for any of us when we move from a private sphere to a public one is to dress and groom ourselves accordingly.

As for Karen, the incident helped her decide to become an electrologist. She had been considering the idea for some months, ever since it had been put to her by the electrologist she herself was seeing twice a week.

Karen had met this electrologist after what she refers to as the most embarrassing night of her life. 'I'd curled up in bed with a man I'd just made love to,' explained Karen, 'and he put the sheet in between us. I had hair on my stomach and I used to shave it. I guess I must have been scratchy that night. Well, I was mortified to see his reaction, and as soon as he left my apartment the following morning, I picked an electrologist out of the yellow pages and made an appointment.'

Karen became friends with the electrologist, who helped her get training and eventually took her on as a partner. After a few years Karen opened her own practice, which has thrived from the start.

WEIGHTY BUSINESS

The manner in which Karen was recruited into her new occupation is not unusual. Professional body remakers quite commonly come from the ranks of those who have suffered personally with the problem they now treat. In some cases, having been a sufferer is actually an official prerequisite for employment.

This is particularly common in the weight-loss industry, as I learned from a woman who owns a Weight Watchers franchise in the Midwest that runs 400 meetings a week and employs almost 500 people. Nearly all of those employees are 'lifetime members' of Weight Watchers, which means they used to be overweight.

'We're in a business in which weight is essential to the integrity of the organisation. We wouldn't have a ghost of a chance in the community if we didn't present proper role models ourselves,' said Eve, who sets aside time at every business meeting in case any members of her staff are experiencing weight problems they want to discuss.

If an employee does gain weight above the prescribed range, Eve prohibits the person from official contact with the public, sets up individual counselling with an experienced group leader or someone from her managerial staff, and requests that the person attend a Weight Watchers group until the necessary pounds are lost.

As of the time I met her, she had never had to fire anyone because of weight. Those who had been unable to shed the required number of pounds had resigned on their own. But she worried she may someday be sued on grounds of discrimination. 'It's a very sensitive issue around the office,' she said.

Eve, who wears her long black hair in a Gloria Steinem cut, is 43, close to six feet tall, lean, and herself a lifetime member of Weight Watchers. 'My weight problem started when I was 20,' she told me early in our dinner at an elegant restaurant. 'For the first ten years I handled it by starving part of the time and bingeing the rest. By the time I turned 30, I couldn't do that anymore. I couldn't go without eating because I'd get dizzy.

'So I started putting on a lot of weight. I felt like an elephant. I tried everything. I went to the doctors, I tried the liquid protein diet, which made me lose my hair. I took diet pills. Each of them worked for a little while, but not very long. I was on what we call in the weight-loss business the yo-yo syndrome, which can be more detrimental to the human body than carrying extra weight.

'Eventually I joined Weight Watchers, and believe me, I was one of the biggest sceptics who ever walked into the room. Number one, they were telling me to eat food, which I figured couldn't possibly work. If *not* eating wasn't working, how could eating work?'

Rather than counting calories, Weight Watchers provides menus that include precise portions of fruits, vegetables, dairy products, and meat, fish or poultry. The member is required to eat three substantial meals a day and a snack.

'I was sceptical, but I promised myself that I would do what they told me,' she went on, narrating a story she had no doubt recounted many times in the ten years since she lost 29 pounds, but one she told with obvious relish. 'So I got the programme, went home, and for the first time in my life, I cooked. I'd never been in the kitchen before, but here I was taking pains to cook properly. I weighed everything as they told me to, and I ate everything they allowed me to eat, which was volumes more than I'd been eating.'

At this point we were interrupted by the waiter. We both ordered the broiled swordfish and mixed green salad, and Eve continued her story.

'They don't allow you to weigh yourself between meetings, because if

you lose weight you'll reward yourself with food and gain back everything you lost. So I showed up the next week absolutely *certain* I'd gained
five pounds. I was so embarrassed. I went to the meeting in my raincoat.
Actually I'd *lost* two and a half pounds.

'I though it was a fluke. But the next week I lost again, and the next
week again . . . and I got hooked. It gives you something to look forward
to, going to the meeting and weighing in.

'People who haven't had a weight problem just don't understand,' she
continued. 'They look at the person and they think, "How could she let
herself get that way?" They have pat theories about why people are fat,
like assuming that people overeat when they're depressed. Well, sure,
some people eat when they're depressed. And some people eat when
they're happy. Some people eat when they fail, some people eat when they
succeed. There are all different triggers for overeating.'

What is *her* answer to the question of why people get fat, I asked.

'Interestingly,' she replied, 'I've never been asked that before.' She took
a sip of water while framing her answer. 'I imagine there are as many
reasons for someone to be overweight as there are' – looking around the
room for a good comparison – 'recipes for bread. *My* reasons for having
the problem were all emotional. Every emotional high and low caused
me to eat.

'Also, as a child I was constantly given rich food. Ice cream, candy,
cakes. My parents, whom I love very much, weren't doing this maliciously,
since I was reasonably thin at that time. But as I got older and started
gaining weight, I didn't know how to eat.'

Members of Weight Watchers don't make this mistake, she told me.
They learn proper ways to eat and pass these along to their children.

Eve went on to describe what she called the 'magic' of the programme:
the newspaper she publishes every month with 'before' and 'after' pictures
of members who lost 30 or 45 or 85 pounds and look like different
people; the heartwarming letters she receives from people whose lives
have been turned around.

Actually, Eve did not need to sell me on the value of the self-help
method; I consider it one of the great social inventions of this century.
These groups are so successful that professionals ask *them* for assistance
at times – as evidenced by Alcoholics Anonymous chapters within psychiatric hospitals.

The key to the success of self-help groups is an ingenious bit of sleight
of hand they perform. They treat members' weaknesses as assets.
Instead of feeling guilty or hopeless because you went off the wagon or
into an ice cream parlour, you are encouraged to relate those experiences
at group meetings so they might help others.

And if you do succeed at controlling your weight, you may even gain
a job. Eve informed me that over the years her franchise has hired as

group leaders and clerical workers about 1,000 members of the organisation, many of whom had been depressed and unemployable housewives before joining Weight Watchers.

By bringing together people from diverse backgrounds, groups like Weight Watchers accomplish another remarkable feat of social engineering. This Eve called to my attention when I asked her – after the swordfish arrived – to describe the ingredients in an effective Weight Watchers meeting. She immediately pointed to the fact that groups in her territory include blacks and whites, Jews and gentiles, rich and poor, young and old, women and men.

'Newcomers walk into that room with a lot of pain and guilt, and what do they see? They see they are not alone. Even though their problem may take on a different tone, all the people in that room, regardless of how much money they make or how wonderful they look now, have the same problem.

'It becomes a real family in that meeting room. You don't sit in a meeting for an hour and a half and just think about how many pounds you've lost. You start to listen. You go in thinking you're unique, you're the only one who has starved and not lost weight, who can't control her appetite. Then you hear the other people, and you feel all the support there is among people who have a common problem.'

Another reason why a 'family' feeling develops in these sorts of groups is that people who lose weight often discover that the real family and friends are less than supportive. When someone commits to change, friends are likely to feel threatened. Eve, who led groups herself for several years, told me that a great deal of time is spent in Weight Watchers meetings discussing the reactions of family and friends.

'People who lose weight,' she said, 'do more than lose weight. They go through a transformation. Very often, those you consider your closest friends don't like seeing you looking that good. They tend to get jealous or angry.' Eve estimated that about half the members who lose weight and keep it off also lose a close friendship in the process, or a marriage.

Yet the problems that members experience in their personal lives are off-limits in Weight Watchers meetings. Eve said her group leaders are instructed to stick as closely as possible to the topic, of how to eat properly.

'We never get away from why we're there,' she said, wagging her fork at me as if reprimanding one of her staff. 'We're not in the psychology business. We are not therapists. A Weight Watchers meeting is not a therapy session. It is not a bull session, and it's not a gripe session.'

What if someone comes in and says, 'I had a big fight with my spouse, so I had a bad week,' what do you say to that person? I asked.

'What did you do?' she said to me as if I were the member in question.

I overate, I said.

'What did you eat?'

Two chocolate cream pies and a gallon of ice cream in two days.

'Susie,' Eve said to an imaginary person at the table next to ours, 'what could Barry have done? How could he have used that time constructively for himself?' Turning to me and smiling warmly: 'How did it make you feel to eat that stuff? I'm so glad you came to the meeting tonight, Barry. You really needed the meeting, and you felt good enough about yourself to come even though you didn't have a great week. But this coming week's going to be better.'

I pushed the point: You won't talk about the conflict with the spouse at all?

'Absolutely not. We're not equipped.' She paused just long enough to anticipate my next question. 'If your point is that we're not dealing with the *real* problem, I say poppy-cock. We're dealing with the overeating problem. The marital problem is a different problem. If the fight with the partner is around eating, there are specific kinds of helpful ideas that can come from other members in the room about dealing with discouragers.'

The guiding principle in such instances, Eve explained, is that people criticise you because they themselves are hurting. Quite likely, they are unhappy with their own weight. So the best response is just to let them vent those feelings without becoming defensive or angry in return.

Maybe so. But might there not be another reason for some friends and spouses to react negatively to a Weight Watchers convert? Perhaps, I suggested to Eve, they do not understand the person's new ways of thinking and behaving or they feel left out because the person has a new 'family'.

Eve's rejoinder was that this is just another example of how people stereotype overweight people. If they do nothing about their fat, they're considered lazy or stupid, employers discriminate against them and they are forced to buy clothes in special stores. Yet if they slim down, some will say they have given up their real selves or become zealots. Hogwash, said Eve.

Good point, said I, finishing the last of my fish. But now that she had brought up the matter of prejudice against the obese, another question came to mind. Doesn't Weight Watchers itself put forward a message that it is bad or pitiable to be heavy? The co-founder of Weight Watchers, Albert Lippert, has been quoted as saying 'It's simple, really. Fat people are not happy' (Lippert, 1978: 100).

While this is a popular assumption about the obese, recent surveys, I indicated to Eve, suggest it is inaccurate. Overweight adults are no more anxious or depressed than others, one study found (Hayes and Ross, 1986). Another found that 49 per cent of women and 55 per cent of men who consider themselves overweight said they feel good about their appearance none the less (Cash *et al.*, 1986).

Eve took another tack. 'We're not saying it's *bad*,' she said, 'we're saying it's unhealthful. There are healthful weights listed on the Metropolitan Life Insurance tables. Those are the weights at which you live optimally.'

Like other body remakers I have interviewed, Eve wants to hide behind the shibboleth called Health. She claims that her programme makes it possible for some people to live longer and have fewer illnesses; and this benefit far outweighs any unintended harm the programme might cause those who choose not to join, or who join but do not succeed.

That argument would be more compelling were it not for the conspicuous lack of consensus among scientists on these matters. Several leading authorities contend, for instance, that half or more of the obese population would be better off fat than suffer the physiological and psychological problems that accompany their efforts to diet. And some studies indicate that the healthiest people weigh 15 to 20 pounds more than the famous Metropolitan Life tables say they should (Cahnman, 1968; Andres, 1980; Ritenbaugh, 1982; Brody, 1987).

Not that the notion of optimal weights is entirely lacking in merit. The numbers on the Metropolitan Life tables are certainly superior to the other leading point of reference available in our culture: namely, the ideal images in the media. Weight Watchers authorises people to feel good about their bodies while remaining considerably heavier than the official beauties they see in the magazines and on television. And Eve's employees can lose their jobs for falling *below* the specified range for their age and height, as well as for rising above.

Still, use of the weight tables results in the exclusion of some people who may want or need the services of Weight Watchers. A member who is unable (or does not wish) to lose the required number of pounds by means of the programme's menu prescriptions is not permitted to enter the second phase of the programme, the weight-maintenance classes. Even those who function well and are happy at higher weights are not eligible for classes that could help them stay at their preferred weight, nor can they become lifetime members.

When I raised this matter, Eve found herself unable to offer an argument why such exclusion should be the case. 'People who look better feel better,' she said, 'and people who feel better function better.' I reminded her that I have interviewed people who have discovered through trial and error that they feel and function best when their weight is well above what the tables deem normal.

'To be perfectly blunt,' she eventually conceded, 'we wouldn't have much of a business if people were running around saying they're lifetime members of Weight Watchers when they're eighty pounds overweight.'

PLASTIC MONEY

The not-so-secret truth about body remaking is that it is as much about big business as it is about improved health. Americans spend $10 billion annually on diet programmes and products. Between its classes and food products, Weight Watchers alone is nearly a billion-dollar-a-year enterprise, and a large franchise like Eve's can gross $5 million.

Although Weight Watchers has 75 per cent of the US market for weight-loss lessons, that still leaves room for several huge competitors. For instance, The Diet Centre, a franchise operation with 2,000 outlets nationally that offer individualised counselling and specialised diets in addition to group classes, racks up revenues in the $40 million range.

The national market for weight loss is truly gargantuan. According to surveys, 55 per cent of women and 41 per cent of men believe they are overweight, and 65 million Americans are dieting.[2] And people who consider themselves overweight tend to be repeat customers for the diet industry. The vast majority of dieters try many programmes during their lifetimes – only 5 to 10 per cent of those who lose weight manage to keep it off for more than two years. As a result, diet programmes are constantly advertising in an effort to steal one another's members, and to pick up those who have given up on their current programme.

Much as the existence of a massive defence industry ensures that the nation will build more and more weapons, the sheer size of the diet industry guarantees that we'll buy additional weight-loss products. Supply helps to produce demand. In both cases, the industries pump a great deal of money into research, advertising and public relations to persuade us that by supporting them we improve our own chances of survival.

Yet the fastest-growing field in body remaking is not weight loss but cosmetic surgery. The number of cosmetic surgery operations performed in the US doubled between 1981 and 1987. Today, 600,000 operations to make people look younger or more beautiful are performed annually.[3]

Women make up the vast majority of cosmetic surgery patients, which is hardly surprising, given the differences in how men and women express vanity and the fact that breast enhancement alone accounts for close to one-fifth of all cosmetic surgeries. Were a biceps augmentation procedure perfected, we might see men swarm into cosmetic surgeons' offices.

Even so, one-third of men in a national survey (as compared to 45 per cent of women) said they would consider having cosmetic surgery. With articles in business magazines singing the praises of cosmetic surgery, the male market is growing, and for some procedures it is already strong. Men account for one-quarter of all nose jobs (rhinoplasties), for example, and nearly one-fifth of eyelid surgeries (blepharoplasties).

In all, cosmetic surgeons rake in about $5 billion a year. Advertising budgets at large cosmetic surgery centres can exceed $1 million a year, for procedures which typically cost $1,000 to $4,000 each. In some cities, though, a nose job can run to $6,000 and a face-lift can set you back $10,000.

And that is just the cosmetic surgeon's share. Spillover from the cosmetic surgery boom is also generating handsome incomes for other categories of body remakers who provide ancillary services. Allison, the beauty-makeover artist, relies upon referrals from cosmetic surgeons for half of her income.

Women who have had their stomachs tucked or their breasts reduced, said Allison, often notice that their faces, which are still full, no longer match the rest of their body. Their cosmetic surgeons send them to Allison's Upper East Side Manhattan studio, where they get a new makeup regimen and hairstyle.

Women who have had face-lifts also come to Allison for help. 'They get their new faces, but they still wear their old makeup,' she explained. 'With a larger face, you can wear more makeup. The filling in of the nose, the building up of the lipline, the camouflage on the cheeks . . . all these things they did before their face-lift to create the illusion of being tighter and thinner. After the surgery, they still apply all that gunk, and it makes them look like harlots.'

Increasingly, the women who come to Allison for these postoperative services are in the thirties and forties, rather than in their fifties and sixties as was the case several years ago. Nationally, over one-third of patients who have face-lifts are younger than 50.

Even though it is good for her business, Allison disapproves of this trend. 'I'm not some sort of moralist,' she said. 'Anything somebody wants to do to herself is okay with me. But most of these girls, all they really need is some simple beauty tips.'

To illustrate, she removed from her shoulder bag a copy of a nationally famous women's magazine, turned to a layout about beauty makeovers, and gave me a concise course on how to look more beautiful. 'I was the makeup artist on that shoot,' she announced, 'and 90 per cent of the difference between the "before" and "after" shots was unbelievably simple. First, I got the girl to smile. A smile makes anyone instantly look ten times better. Then I had her straighten up her posture. If you stand up straight you instantly lose five pounds.

'Then I put a little concealer and some powder to get rid of the dark circles under eyes. She could have paid a plastic surgeon $4,000 to accomplish the same thing. Then I located her cheekbone. You'd be surprised how many women say to me, "I don't *have* a cheekbone." I say, "Trust me, you do have a cheekbone, and you can give the illusion of having a *high* cheekbone by placing your blush under your cheekbone instead of on it or above it." '

'From there on, it's all a matter of drawing attention away from some spots and on to others. If a girl is a little overweight, the first thing I'll do is put some dynamic earrings on her to direct everything to her face.'

If effecting a transformation is so simple, I responded, why are women selecting the cosmetic surgery options instead?

'They're lazy,' said Allison. 'It's easier than learning how to use makeup and accessories properly and working on your face every morning. Why does somebody go to a surgeon for a weight problem instead of eating properly and getting some exercise? It's the same thing.'

Not necessarily. For many people, cosmetic surgery is enticing precisely because they think of it as an active endeavour – as one more piece in a comprehensive health-and-fitness programme.

That is certainly the way cosmetic surgeons are promoting their services. An advertisement for a clinic in California features a photo of an attractive woman, captioned: 'It's important for me to look and feel the best I can. And that's why I eat the right foods and exercise. And that's why I had plastic surgery' (cited in Dull and West (1987)).

This view of cosmetic surgery stands a good chance of winning public acceptance over the next several years, given our tendency to confuse beauty with health. But some cosmetic surgeons are strongly critical of it. In an editorial in a professional journal, Robert Goldwyn (1985), a surgeon from Massachusetts, warned his colleagues 'of an alarming rise of hucksterism, a fearful professional pestilence'. Appalled by a letter another surgeon had mailed to his patients, encouraging them to have excess fat removed and their breasts enlarged or reduced in preparation for the beach season, Goldwyn wrote sarcastically: 'Our surgical Lancelot, thank God, is ready to take up scalpel and suction for the afflicted. I was not surprised that he, so busy to benefit from the beach, did not tell his patients to protect themselves from the sun.'

Other doctors have raised more sober concerns about the healthfulness of operations performed primarily for reasons of vanity. Some complications of cosmetic surgery occur frequently enough, these physicians point out, that they should not be taken lightly; among the most common are scarring, secondary infections, bleeding and skin discoloration. Less common but more frightening are nerve damage and loss of sensation or motor ability (Rosenthal, 1982; Lefton, 1985; Scheiner, 1986).

Public health advocates have suggested that cosmetic surgery is a drain on the nation's health care resources (Williams, 1985; Jones, 1986; Northrup, 1987). Forty per cent of the board-certified physicians who are members of the American Society of Plastic and Reconstructive Surgeons restrict their practices to beautification surgery. Rarely if ever do they perform reconstructive plastic surgery such as emergency-room care, cleft-palate operations, or the repair of injured limbs.

'Fourteen years of expensive medical education to take off wrinkles from somebody's face is a travesty,' said Stuart, a plastic surgeon in

Atlanta, when I raised the topic of cosmetic surgery. 'In this country we are not in a situation comparable to the Third World yet; we're not bankrupt, we can afford these luxuries. Still, it is insane. Where is the justification for helping people to run away from the reality of growing old, when your time could be spent on those who are truly ill?'

Stuart's orientation to his profession is expressed in his office decoration. The only wall hangings are his diplomas; the only artworks a half-dozen clay and plastic sculptures of human hands, breasts and noses scattered among the book-shelves. The focus in the stark white room is his paper-cluttered metal desk and opposite it two chairs intended for patients and the partners.

For our interview I sat in the chair to his left, and Stuart, a heavy-set man with a bulbous nose, was seated behind the desk. 'Too many accident victims and cancer patients in this city need my services for me to spend my time on vanity surgery,' he said fervently.

Not that he is a purist. He does perform some cosmetic surgery, he let me know. It is just that he chooses carefully which patients to take on and restricts the cosmetic part of his practice to one-quarter of his time – 'much to the chagrin of my wife,' he added, 'who for the life of her cannot understand why the Milquetoast dermatologist at the end of our street makes twice what I do.'

How does he decide which applicants for cosmetic surgery to accept, I asked.

'If you're really ageing prematurely and you have deep jowls and neck wrinkles that keep you uncomfortable, wet and macerated in the summers, that's a valid reason,' Stuart replied. 'But to do it because the "in" thing to do this year is to get a face-lift for your 45th birthday, I'm not willing to participate.

'Some major corporations practically make it a condition of employment that senior people have a face-lift or some work done around their eyes. If I'm approached by a reasonable 50–year-old executive who comes in here and says, "Things are tight, I need to look a bit younger and less tired if I'm going to have a chance," I say, fine. It may not be absolutely the right reason for it, but it's reasonable, it's an acceptable reason for him to be asking. Compare that to the woman who comes in saying, "My husband's fooling around, and I've got to get him back." I would turn her away.'

Why should the businessman's request be deemed more reasonable than the wife's? I asked. Isn't that sexist?

'After the face-lift, her marriage is still going to be lousy,' Stuart contended. 'She'll return a month later angry with me. "He still ran away with my neighbour, and I'm going to sue you for all you're worth." It is your job as a physician to decide what are reasonable goals and expectations of a patient.'

The principle Stuart was trying to get across – and the one that guides his medical decision making – is that cosmetic surgery is warranted only when it will improve how a person functions in the world. To illustrate his point, he took a couple of photographs from a drawer.

The first was of a very attractive black woman. 'Here's an example of a woman I did choose to work on. She was a newspaper reporter with ambitions to be in television. She was obviously quite bright – all A's as a student at Emory – and there was little doubt she could succeed in her chosen profession, except that she had exaggerated African features. In a Caucasian-oriented industry, she would not be considered attractive. I pulled her jaw back, narrowed and raised her nose, and sent her to a colleague for some orthodontic work.' He explained that this woman, unlike the wife with the philandering husband, could be helped to function better by means of cosmetic surgery.

Then Stuart picked up the second photograph, but before showing it to me he asked, 'How many fingers does Mickey Mouse have?' Try as I might to remember what Mickey looks like, to figure out why Stuart would be asking me this question, I could not.

'Most people don't realise that Disney characters have only three fingers and a thumb,' he instructed, and showed me the picture he was holding, which was not of Mickey Mouse, but of a human hand with four fingers.

'You can do everything with four fingers you can do with five,' Stuart said. 'The brain switches over right away. And yet accident victims will fight and not be willing to lose even a part of a finger. They'd rather spend their whole lives babying an abnormal part that would have been better off in the bucket so they can look "normal". This reality is, most people they come in contact with won't even notice that they have only four fingers.'

His argument was compelling, and yet I wondered how well one can distinguish between function and aesthetics in actual practice. Maybe the absence of a finger would cause people embarrassment every time they are asked to shake hands, or lose someone a high-paying sales job. Who can say in advance?

Ironically, in the case of cosmetic rather than reconstructive surgery, the line between practicality and beauty may be even harder to draw. We live in a society in which attractiveness brings rewards, and so the odds are good that an operation that makes a person more beautiful will also improve how he or she gets along in the world.

Patients who undergo cosmetic surgery are usually pleased with the results, according to studies, and are perceived by others as more sexually appealing and responsive and as better marriage partners after their operations. One researcher reported improvements in the personalities of fully two-thirds of a sample of patients following cosmetic surgery. Contrary to Stuart's expectations, studies have found that lifting a woman's face or breasts will often boost her spirits and her marriage (Reich, 1969; Berscheid and Gangestad, 1982; Fisher, 1986; Hollyman *et al.*, 1986).

Determining what constitutes an improvement in functioning can be difficult, as I tried to suggest to Stuart by way of the example of a young woman I interviewed. She did well in school and had plenty of friends, but she was preoccupied by the fact that her breasts were larger than any of her friends.

They were not so large that they caused back problems, however, nor did they create difficulties in buying clothes. For those reasons, her family physician refused to give her a referral when she decided to have a breast-reduction operation performed.

By her own account, not much changed in her life after she had the operation, except that she felt less self-conscious, and men on the street stared at her less frequently.

In this case, like many in cosmetic surgery, little improvement in functioning was gained. On the other hand, does this distinguish cosmetic surgery from every other medical speciality? Some allergists make a good chunk of their incomes by administering weekly shots to people whose allergies are not severe enough to handicap them, nor even to cause discomfort for more than a few weeks every year. Often the treatments do not help these people anyway.

'But let's carry your analogy one step further,' said Stuart. 'Granted, people have a natural urge to look normal, just as they do to sneeze in the presence of allergens. But it's getting to the point that we are spreading the infection we're charged with treating.

'How would it be if allergists placed scratch-and-sniff advertisements in magazines, advertisements that contained chemicals that caused readers to react? That is essentially what cosmetic surgeons do.

'Plastic surgeons shouldn't promote the disabling notion that beauty is a valuable end in its own right, any more than oncologists should promote cigarette smoking. I've heard intelligent people come up with good arguments for that one too, by the way. "Smoking reduces stress." "If it helps them keep their weight down, maybe it's not so bad." ' Stuart quoted these comments with a pronounced sneer, but then a sad expression spread across his face.

'I'll tell you a perversely humorous story about the clinical dangers of vanity,' he continued. 'A woman I operated on last week is the mistress of a local physician, an internist. She had a 10–centimetre tumour in her breast. Malignant. He claims he didn't notice it.

'How could he not notice it? I could believe that maybe someone, even a doctor, would overlook a tumour in his *wife's* breast, but how he could fail to notice one in his *mistress's* breast is beyond me. I guess he wasn't thinking of her breasts in any manner except as objects for his sexual pleasure.

'But then', he added, 'she wasn't much better in that regard herself. The day she came to my office, she was wearing a low-neck dress and had put makeup on her cleavage to hide the age lines. This was after an oncologist had found nineteen positive nodes under her arm, in addition to those in her breast, and told her she'd have to have major surgery.'

PLAYBOY AS A TAX DEDUCTION

Stuart's receptionist interrupted us at this point with the news that we had gone over time and patients were waiting. He had one more point he wanted to make, though, before I left, and to do so he took out another visual aid from his desk. It was the current issue of *Playboy*, which seemed out of place in this austere office.

'The Saks Fifth Avenue catalogue of our profession,' he said, holding the magazine in front of him. 'If you want to know which breast shape is stylish this year, just open up and look. Want to determine whether we're going with Irish turned-up noses this season or the Swedish bob?'

There was anger in Stuart's voice.

'It is travesty enough that our profession actively promotes vanity. On top of that, we practice inferior aesthetics. A woman can walk into a cosmetic surgeon's office – a thin woman of Mediterranean ancestry, let us say – and ask for a northern European nose and 38 inch breasts. If her credit rating checks out, the surgeon will comply with her request, even though her face will look asinine as a result, and her figure will be all out of proportion.

'There are objective procedures one can use in plastic surgery. With a rhinoplasty, for instance, you measure the vertical height of the face, how much projection the chin has, the space between the eyes, the relative location of the cheekbone. Then you build a nose that will blend in with the other features.

'For a patient who seeks a simple rhinoplasty to remove a bump or straighten out a crooked nose, these kinds of considerations are all that come into play. They should be in every other case as well, but try to tell that to a Jewish mother who brings you her daughter and a photograph of Brooke Shields and demands that you fit the kid with a schnozz like the one in the picture.'

He thumped the copy of *Playboy* on his desktop. 'The IRS has ruled that a subscription to *Playboy* magazine is a tax-deductible expense for a plastic surgeon. And frankly, I cannot honestly dispute the ruling. It's a tool of the trade in some practices.'

Stuart's comments point up the extent to which bodies themselves have become objects to be sold in American society. Surgeons sell not just corrections to the body – to make us look more normal or attractive – but something far more transitory, *fashions*. They alter the size and shape of our buttocks, breasts, noses, or eyes to fit current styles.

If the period from the mid-1800s to the mid-1900s was one in which the individual's body became a vehicle for the display of consumer products, lately we are faced with the next logical step in consumerism. No longer can we merely dress up the body we happen to have, or improve it by losing weight or having a beauty makeover or straightening out the curve in our nose. We must actually purchase a 'new body'.

In a literal sense, of course, it is impossible to trade in our bodies for new ones. Even if a cosmetic surgeon altered every region of our anatomy, the best we would end up with is a revamped version of the body we were born with. The crucial point is rather that so many people *think* in terms of getting a new body that it makes sense these days to *talk* in those terms. Where else but in modern-day America could a magazine titled *New Body* find an audience?

The mounting enthusiasm for cosmetic surgery actually represents only the most glaring evidence for this latest view of the body. The notion of gaining a new body is most highly developed elsewhere – within the contemporary fitness movement.

If cosmetic surgeons offer to change our looks and, as a consequence, our prospects for love or wealth, those who promote exercise hold out all that and more. They say the new body that results from proper exercise will keep us alive longer, save money for our employers and raise our social status.

NOTES

1 This is an edited version of a chapter from *Bodies: Overcoming the Tyranny of Perfection* first published in the USA in 1992, which the author, sociologist Barry Glassner, has kindly agreed to let us publish here. It provides an entertaining and insightful introduction to the nature of health-related consumer culture in the USA and as such provides an analysis of tendencies already apparent within a British context [eds].
2 Information from H. J. Heinz Co. (owner of Weight Watchers). See also the data in Fannin (1986), Kleinfield (1986) and Cash *et al.* (1986).
3 Information from the American Society of Plastic and Reconstructive Surgeons. See also Cash *et al.* (1986) and Kaplan (1986).

Chapter 14

Positive ageing

What is the message?

Mike Hepworth

INTRODUCTION

One aspect of health promotion as it has emerged in the late twentieth century is the concern to establish a relationship between health, healthy living and positive ageing into old age. Attempts to establish connections between lifestyle and health have resulted in increasing attention being paid to the adult ageing process and techniques for combatting the more deleterious consequences of biological ageing in later life. The concept of 'positive ageing' therefore focuses attention on an issue which is of interest both to sociologists of health promotion and social gerontologists: namely, the emerging tendency to construct *moral* distinctions between styles of ageing and old age, and it is this aspect of the conjunction between health promotion and social gerontology that is the subject of this chapter.

But first it is necessary to spell out the usage of the term 'moral' in this discussion. Two interpretations of the concept of moral are employed: first, in the conventional ethical sense with reference to distinctions between right and wrong, virtuous and non-virtuous; and, second, in the sociological interpretation of 'moral' established by Goffman (1968a; 1968b) to refer to changes in the expression of social identity as individuals move through everyday life from one social situation and status to another. Goffman argued for an extension of the scope of the concept of 'career' from its narrower conventional reference to progress in a 'respectable profession' (Goffman, 1968a: 119) to include 'any social strand of any person's course through life' (1968a: 119). As a universal process of potential transition and change throughout the life course, moral aspects of the career process include 'the regular sequence of changes that career entails in the person's self and in his (*sic*) framework of imagery for judging himself (*sic*) and others' (Goffman, 1968a: 119). Such processes of self-judgement are morally grounded in the fact that every society 'establishes the means of categorising persons and the complement of attributes felt to be ordinary and natural for members of each of these categories' (Goffman, 1968b: 11). In this sociological model the two conceptions of moral are thus interconnected: the 'moral career' of the self through life derives its structure and meaning from moral conceptions of what is normal and socially acceptable in any given prescribed category. In short, social categorisation is essentially a process of moral categorisation.

Following this line of sociological analysis, it is argued that given the acknowledged existence of variations in the processes of biological ageing (Krauss Whitbourne, 1985), positive and negative styles of ageing into old age are not objectively distinctive physical conditions waiting to be discovered once the appropriate medico-scientific methodology has been refined, but are socially constructed moral categories reflecting the prevailing social preference for individualised consumerism, voluntarism and decentralisation. It is argued that these social preferences foster an accelerating age-consciousness where the fear of ageing into old age tends to predominate, and old age is consequently perceived as a 'social problem' which can only be resolved by normalising styles of ageing prescriptively designated 'positive' (i.e. as the bodily evidence of 'rational' and independent individual lifestyles), and discouraging or even punishing styles of ageing defined as deviant (i.e. 'irrational', self-indulgent and, above all, conducive to social dependency).

POSITIVE AGEING

The dictionary defines one of the key meanings of the word 'positive' as: 'of an affirmative nature', 'definite', 'confident'. Positive is, of course, the direct opposite of 'negative'. In direct contrast, the word 'negative' means 'a thing whose essence consists in the absence of something positive' (Oxford Universal Dictionary, 1965).

In the literature of social gerontology the word 'positive' is conventionally deployed with reference to the importance of encouraging or developing a 'positive attitude' towards ageing into old age. For example, Tinker's textbook, *Elderly People in Modern Society* (1992) endorses the appeal for what Keddie, a consultant psychiatrist, is quoted as describing as 'positive thinking' about ageing and old age. The familiar argument is rehearsed that a great deal of the discussion of this subject is 'inappropriately negative, pessimistic and too often couched in crisis terms' (Tinker, 1992: 9). Such negative terminology is conventionally, and correctly, attributed in the literature of social gerontology to the pernicious influence of ageism or prejudice against older people collectively stereotyped as a section of the population disqualified by reason of their chronological age from making a full contribution to society.

The term 'ageism' first came to light in America when Robert Butler used what he originally described as 'Age-Ism' to identify wholesale discrimination against all older people which, he argued, rivalled racism 'as the great issue of the next 20 to 30 years' (Butler, 1969: 246) and thus represented a major barrier to their welfare and to the understanding of later life. Since that time academic gerontologists, pressure groups, and professional workers have been drawn to a common cause: the struggle against ageism in contemporary society. 'Ageism', writes Biggs 'is now established, amongst gerontologists at least, as a starting point for nearly all investigations of older age' (Biggs, 1993: 86). The conventional geron- tological wisdom is that prejudice against ageing and old age, as reflected in negative stereotypes of the ageing process as essentially decremental, is a pervasive evil that must be eliminated in a world in which the population is rapidly growing older. Health professionals too are now beginning to include the battle against ageism in their definition of the nature and scope of health promotion as a process of enabling 'positive health – comprising well-being and fitness' (Health Education Board For Scotland, 1992: 3) through the encouragement of individual responsibility for the maintenance of a positive lifestyle.

Writing, for example, in the context of the problem of ageing into old age in Ireland, Kelleher (1993) cites ageism as the legitimate target of those concerned with the promotion of 'personal health and wellbeing' (Kelleher, 1993: 13). Ageism, defined once again as 'the widespread (negative) stereotyping of people because they are old' (Kelleher, 1993: 42), acts as a barrier to equitable health promotion because it prevents the recognition of older people as capable of taking a positive attitude towards the influence of lifestyle on health and therefore the ageing process. It is important to acknowledge that most older people are rela- tively healthy and that, significantly, their preventive practices are 'gener- ally equal to or better than those of younger people' (Kelleher, 1993: 48). Older people in general are therefore fully 'capable of acting upon health promotion advice about factors such as diet, exercise and smoking. This is despite the fact that their habits earlier in life may not have been particularly "healthy" ' (Kelleher, 1993: 48). One of the primary aims of health promotion is to rescue older people from the marginal regions of society and to reconstruct them as the active consumers of health promotion techniques including 'preparation for ageing, health mainten- ance and lifestyle modification, personal skills development and social change to facilitate health' (Kelleher, 1993: 13).

A specific example of the attempt to confront the negative attitudes associated with the deleterious effects of ageism on the health and well- being of older people can be found in H. B. Gibson's manual, *The Emotional and Sexual Lives of Older People* (1992). In this pioneering study the author advocates the positive encouragement of emotional and sexual expression in later life: 'Throughout life most people need to regard themselves positively with regard to their feminine or masculine sexuality. This is generally a deep psychological need, and denial of it may lead to depression and preternatural ageing' (Gibson, 1992: 173) (it is worth recalling that the word 'preternatural' means 'out of the ordinary course of nature' (Oxford Universal Dictionary, 1992: 1,965)). 'We have', Gibson writes, 'discussed the stereotypes of the elderly as currently held by both professional and lay people, and it seems that although there is a growing liberalisation of attitudes, we have a very long way to go yet in approaching anything like a reasonable view of ageing as an acceptable process in everyone's life' (Gibson, 1992: 77). Although he does not make explicit use of the term 'positive', ageing that allows a full range of adult emotional and sexual expression can be described as 'positive', whereas ageing that is essentially a repressive hangover from our Victorian past, and which should therefore be discarded as soon as possible, may be described as 'negative'. For Gibson positive ageing is the recommended reconstituted norm and its opposite, negative ageing, is relegated to the deviant fringe.

In any sociological analysis of the substance and interdependencies of concepts of positive and negative attitudes towards ageing and old age it is important to emphasise that their theory and practice is not confined to the professionals. In a paper, 'Who Theorises Age?', Gubrium and Brandon Wallace (1990) argue that theorising about growing older is not only the activity of 'professional social gerontologists' but a universal aspect of everyday life 'to the extent that we set about the task of attempting to understand the whys and wherefores of growing old' (Gubrium and Brandon Wallace, 1990: 132). Evidence of the widespread nature of everyday theorising about ageing makes it necessary, they suggest, for scientific gerontologists to incorporate such theories into their technical frame of reference and models of ageing. It may be added that if we follow this advice we discover evidence in empirical research into the day-to-day experiences of growing older that much of the theorising of ordinary men and women is essentially moral in its perspective on the relationships between individual lifestyles, physical health and the maintenance of an independent old age.

In what has become one of the classic participant-observation studies of the adaptations of older people (mostly men and a number of women) living in 'single room occupancies' (SRO) in a slum hotel, the 'Guinevere', in a large American Midwestern city, Stephens (1980) recorded the continuous efforts made by ageing tenants to preserve their individuality and independence in a predatory and deviant social world. As other researchers in quite different social contexts have confirmed, the basic struggle against the impositions of the ageing body was explicitly a moral one: 'dependency', Stephens emphasises, 'was despised as a cardinal sin in the SRO world' (1980: 98). Physically deteriorating individuals (and it must be noted that health problems were endemic) in a physically deteriorating area of this inner city were anxious to maintain their physical activities as long as possible. The problem, the ' "real problem", as one of her informants put it, "is health" ' (Stephens, 1980: 47). The common factor uniting the highly competitive individuals interviewed was their definition of physical and mental decrements 'as powerfully threatening events that may result in the loss of independence and the erosion of all that they value. This pervasive fear leads to a continual interest in drawing comparisons, in checking up on one's own mental and physical competencies by contrasting them with the sometimes visible and rapid decline of other aged tenants in the hotel' (Stephens, 1980: 41). The preservation of self involves skills of impression management and face-saving that include the creating of a self-enhancing personal biography and 'self-defining to prove oneself superior to the other residents of the Guinevere' (Stephens, 1980: 57).

In a completely different geographical and social world, the city of Aberdeen in the late 1970s, Williams (1990) also concluded that ageing was a moral enterprise. His evidence was drawn from a qualitative study of 70 men and women aged 60 and over with additional reference to random sample data of 619 people from middle- and working-class backgrounds. He discovered that part of the Aberdonian version of the 'Protestant Legacy' inherited by his informants was a set of coherent theories about the normal stages of the ageing process. A central feature was the division of later life into two stages: 'early old age' and 'late old age' (Williams, 1990: 72). The first stage was marked out by retirement and the second in terms of the acknowledgement and ultimate acceptance of the signs of the final deterioration of the body. For these older Aberdonians it was a moral duty to resist the final onset of the signs of ill health and thus 'late old age' as long as was reasonably possible: 'Whatever their disagreements, retirement – the first stage of ageing – carried for Aberdonians an obligation to be active; and they seldom expressed, in the context of early old age, the idea that standards could now be relaxed' (Williams, 1991: 66). A relaxation in the duty to remain active was not morally acceptable; the only justification for reduced activity and social disengagement was the recognisable onset of serious ill health. Significantly Williams notes that 'late old age' was perceived as 'old age proper' because it was 'always in some way external to the person' (1990: 71). Literally speaking, it became legitimate to abandon the struggle against the ageing process when it was perceived that there was nothing in this world left to do. At the same time it is important to add that although

> many people accepted that it was legitimate for the very old to sink into passivity, there remained some who were convinced that resistance in some form was always possible. The most vigorous recommendations

for staving off the second stage of old age were essentially versions of the recommendations ... for preserving (during early old age) resistance against illness. Vigour was sustained by keeping up normal interests and activities, decay was courted by sitting down and doing nothing.

(Williams, 1990: 71)

The contrast between the social contexts of Williams' and Stephens' research could scarcely be greater yet both studies demonstrate the existence of coherent moral theories of the relationship between the maintenance of the body and the persistence of the normal social self. Clear moral distinctions are made between positive and negative attitudes to ageing into old age which are frequently expressed in the form of judgements passed against those who fail to conform to these exacting standards. As sociologists of social deviance have frequently observed, the measure of one's own claim to virtue is the perceived absence in the other of the appropriate admirable qualities.

This view receives further substantiation in the ethnographic study carried out by Jerrome (1992) in 1985 of social relations among members of a number of clubs for older people living in 'Seatown' on the south coast of England. 'Old age', she writes in her discussion of beliefs about ageing, 'is a moral category' (Jerrome, 1992: 142).

Responses to it are a matter of virtue and moral strength or weakness. To be happy and make the best of things in spite of pain and hardship is a moral and social obligation attached to the status of the old or handicapped person. Those who fail are blameworthy, and tend to blame themselves.

(Jerrome, 1992: 142)

Those who experience a sense of self-righteousness are those who cling to what Jerrome describes as the 'resistance model' of ageing. This model is one that 'provides an explanation for failure and unhappiness in the principle of just desserts: "you get out of life what you put into it"' (1992: 142).

Whilst the people studied by Stephens were competitive individualists, often with deviant backgrounds and histories, the subjects of Jerrome's analysis were members of mutually supportive group associations. Their social relationships had therefore a significant part to play in the maintenance of positive attitudes towards the ageing body. A significant difference can also be found in the fact that, as has been already noted, the majority of Stephens' subjects were men; women tend not to pass 'the final period of their lives' (Stephens, 1980: 9) in single room occupancies of slum hotels. The people Jerrome observed and interviewed were for the most part women, many of whom were not surprisingly widowed, although as she emphasises at the beginning of her book, 'for the most part the issues are presented as those of old age as such' (Jerrome, 1992: 4).

The moral struggle of ageing into old age, typical of the members of Jerrome's clubs, was focused, as in the case of Williams' study, upon the body and its perceived health status. Her subjects were preoccupied with negotiating the boundary between active and therefore independent later life and the final stage of justified inactive dependency. Health was defined as a moral standard maintained through the exercise of 'sensible routines and positive attitudes' (Jerrome, 1992: 103). The causes of illness and incapacity (the markers of the status passage to old age) were believed to be partly found at least in the failure to take the appropriate self-protecting evasive action. There was a tendency in the social world discovered by Jerrome to stigmatise the sick and the disabled and thus to disqualify them from what Goffman described as 'full social acceptance' (Goffman, 1968b: 9). Dependency, typified in terms of an unequal balance of power, only became acceptable when an individual had made all reasonable efforts to keep active. Much of the talk in the clubs was concerned with health and illness not because these older people were morbidly preoccupied with their bodies but precisely because it was essential for them to monitor the changes in their bodies and the social and personal implications of these changes. To talk about one's symptoms was to be involved in a process of negotiation over the norms of ageing and old age: by means of 'the comparison of symptoms and responses to them, individuals collectively derive a standard against which to measure their own performance and evaluate other people's' (Jerrome, 1992: 98).

OLD AGE AS A SOCIAL PROBLEM

In her inaugural lecture as Professor of Social Gerontology at the University of Wales, Bangor, Clare Wenger concluded on a note of dismay. 'It has', she said, 'always been a source of frustration to me that the increasing numbers of people who live into old age in the United Kingdom are defined as a social problem rather than as an achievement of the late 20th century' (Wenger, 1993: 19). In this lecture Wenger did not go into any great detail about the nature of the perception of old age as a social problem nor did she enlarge on the sociological characteristics of social problems as such. But it is well worth asking what the sociology of social problems, as it was developed during the 1960s and 1970s, may tell us about emerging attitudes towards ageing during the 1990s.

Between the 1960s and the 1970s the sociology of social problems emerged, as a close relation of the sociology of deviance, in direct opposition to the view that social problems were the sole result of natural and unavoidable causes or of the existence of pervasive forces of evil. In place of such misleading assumptions, it was argued, the question, 'when told something is a social problem', should be asked: "problematic to whom?" ' (Cohen, 1973: 12), thus drawing attention to the role of interest groups and processes of social control in the creation of a social problem. In his textbook *Social Pathology*, Lemert (1951) had argued for a conceptual distinction between, for example, the biological and social factors involved in the recognition of a particular behaviour as socially problematic. He described this distinction as one between 'primary' and 'secondary' deviancy. He argued that biological factors (here we can add processes of biological ageing) could not explain the existence of a social problem because they contained no description of the causal connections between the biological and the structure and functions producing social behaviour. The significant variables were, he proclaimed, socio-psychological in nature.

For Lemert 'primary deviation' was 'polygenetic', arising out of a 'variety of social, cultural, psychological and physiological factors', whilst 'secondary deviation' consisted of 'a special class of socially defined responses which people make to problems created by the social reaction to their deviance' (Lemert, 1967: 40). He went to great pains to stress that the problems created by the reactions of others to a perceived deviation were 'essentially moral problems' (1967: 40), by which he meant 'problems which revolve around stigmatisation, punishments, segregation and social control' (1967: 40). As a result of the application of a moral judgement the secondary deviant is the one whose behaviour has been labelled socially problematic and who, as a further consequence, organises his or her life and selfhood around the negative reactions of others. Echoing Goffman's analysis of the effects of stigmatisation on the moral adaptation of the individual self (Goffman, 1968b), Lemert asserted the role of 'categorical societal definitions which depict polarised moral opposites, and also that self definitions or identities are integral in the sense that individuals respond to themselves as moral types' (Lemert, 1967: 41). Lemert's central contribution to the sociology of social problems can be found therefore in the emphasis he placed upon the processes through which 'public and private agencies actively define and classify people, impose punishments, restrict or open access to rewards and satisfactions, set limits to social interaction, and induct deviants into special, segregated environments' (Lemert, 1967: 41).

Following the sociology of deviancy and social problems in 1979, Miller, a social gerontologist, raised the question of the role of processes of social stigmatisation in later life. Defining ageing as 'a stage in human development in which the biological equipment loses its previous resiliency' (Miller, 1979: 283), he argued that a stage was reached where social factors may come to predominate over the biological. Thus although ageing undoubtedly was a biological process 'the idea of ageing is not'

(1979: 284). Social ageing, he argued, was an ascribed social status and as such was 'both analytically independent from physical ageing and peculiarly subject to being construed as deviance' (1979: 289). Social ageing is a peculiarly appropriate subject for deviancy theory because it is subject to a high degree of social scrutiny and evaluation. Unlike some other forms of deviation it is extremely difficult to conceal.

In a subsequent paper published in 1987 Miller enlarged on his theme. Three types of deviance could be associated with the ageing role: illegitimate (stigmatised); conditionally legitimate; and unconditionally legitimate. Although a person may not be held responsible for his or her behaviour (an example Miller used was retirement) 'we find little or no moral neutrality' (Miller, 1987: 145). There were, he wrote,

> exhortations on every side, revealing a multitude of concerns – how best to prepare for retirement, the appropriate age at which to retire, concern about how to use it, worry about a 'roleless' or meaningless existence during this period (which, it is pointed out, may indeed hasten illness or death), costs and benefits, how to prepare for death and dying, and new employment roles (thus vitiating the very idea of retirement). All of these concerns which are put forth by a veritable army of social agents, educators, economists, and politicians may certainly have their own validity. The intention here is not to discount this validity but to emphasise the degree to which our society imputes social and moral meanings even to unconditionally legitimate behaviours in the ageing role.
>
> (Miller, 1987: 145–6)

What Miller meant, of course, was that the potential loss of function in later life leads to greater likelihood of socially deviant conduct and also that the role and status losses of ageing lead to a general stigmatisation. Stigmatisation, as Goffman showed, implies a moral deficiency and is applied as a means of social control, and in old age there are a number of behaviours for which a person is not held technically responsible but which run counter to dominant moral values. Miller classified eighteen types of deviance that contribute to the concept of social ageing, amongst which he included occasional memory lapses, disrobing behaviour, incontinence, insanitary home making, mistakes in business affairs, argumentativeness, withdrawal and role reversal in relation to adult children.

In the context of an analysis of the history of social policy towards older people in Britain between 1890 and 1976 Macintyre (1976) also argued that any inclination to define old age as a social problem was not the consequence of any observable changes in the actual numbers of older people in the population or their physical and social condition. Such a tendency could more accurately be analysed as a response to fluctuations in attitudes towards older people, which in turn reflected changes in political and socio-economic priorities. Evidence could be discovered of both changes over time in the perception of old age as a social problem and also changes over time in the kind of problem old age was considered to be. In addressing this important issue she isolated two distinctive formulations of old age as a social problem, differences that were in fundamental conflict with one another: namely, the humanitarian evaluation of later life which prescribes community intervention to alleviate the decrements associated with old age, and the organisational where the priorities of social organisations as distinct from the perceived needs of older people tend to predominate. Pursuing this line of analysis, Macintyre divided the years 1890–1978 into three distinctive periods. First, the period 1890–1910, during which there was evidence of an increased concern over the welfare of older people followed by a waning of this concern until the 1940s. Second, the 1940s-1950s: a period of social reconstruction that included the revival of concern about the problem of old age; and third, the 1970s where she detected signs of a resurgence of interest in old age and the early traces of a trend which we are now aware has, during the ensuing years, become more firmly established.

The third period, in the midst of which Macintyre wrote her paper, has seen a rapid expansion in social gerontology and the reconstruction of later life through the elaboration of new life 'stages' and transitions. As Jerrome has noted, one of the key developments during these more recent years has been the construction of a distinction 'between early and late stages of old age' involving the encouragement of social scientists to study

> the process by which a person becomes 'old' and is labelled 'old'. Most recently, theoretical interest has shifted from the refinement of age categories to the point of transition from one life phase to the next. Attention has been focused on the boundary situation and the strategies adopted by individuals in their attempt to avoid or hasten upgrading ... The study of the way in which age roles are defined, learned and sustained – in a word, socially constructed – is legitimated by the allocation of public funds, perhaps the final step in the process of institutionalisation.
>
> (Jerrome, 1992: 5)

New norms are therefore being created through the reconstruction of what in earlier times was regarded as an amorphous 'old age' and new norms, of course, imply new forms of deviation and of social sanction.

It is at this point that the parallels between contemporary social gerontology and developments in the sociology of crime and deviance in the 1960s and 1970s become relevant. Following the sociologists of social problems, it can be argued that distinctions between positive and negative ageing into old age are created and elaborated in a social context of increasing concern over the ageing of the population in a society where increasing emphasis is also placed upon the dependence of full social membership and self-validation on a physically active biological body. Moral evaluations of the primacy of the active body in later life – of the virtuous nature of 'keeping right on to the end of the road' – are mutually reinforcing at the micro and macro levels of social organisation.

Social problems theory proposes that collective fear plays a significant role in the creation of a social problem and the fear of ageing (as revealed for example in ageist imagery and behaviour (Featherstone and Hepworth, 1993)) is especially urgent because it refers to important questions about the ironic limitations imposed by the human body. As Kathleen Woodward (1991) argues in her study of representations of old age in twentieth century literature, this question is one that is deeply repressed in contemporary thought. The prevailing fear of ageing has a deeply entrenched cultural history. For the most part images of ageing and old age have reflected widespread anxiety and fear and have provoked denial and repression. She insists that

> old age is a time in our lives about which many of us feel anxiety and fear. The symptoms of these feelings of apprehension are denial and repression of the very subject of ageing and old age. But a fear of ageing is not strictly speaking a 'personal' problem. Our culture's representations of ageing are predominantly negative and thus are inextricably linked to our personal anxieties – for ourselves and for others.
>
> (Woodward, 1991: 4)

In advanced old age, Woodward argues, the most important 'difference' that distinguishes our bodies from those of others is the opposition between youth and age: 'For all of us, if we live long enough, that difference is constructed as old age' (Woodward, 1991: 16). Yet for Woodward old age is not an empty space waiting to be occupied by a positive image. There are limits to constructionism: 'we are', she argues, 'unable to adopt a position of pure social constructivism' (1991: 18) to the ageing body.

> The inevitable and literal association of advanced old age with increasing frailty and ultimately death itself presents a limit beyond which we cannot go. The body in advanced old age not only represents death; it is close to death and will in due time be inhabited by death. The facticity of the mortal vulnerability of the body in old age, and the meanings we attach to it, cannot be explained away by insisting that an ideology of youth, with its corresponding semiotics, is responsible for negative representations of old age.
>
> (Woodward, 1991: 19)

As a consequence,

> however much we may wish to construct alternative representations of ageing for our culture and for ourselves, it remains true in the West, if not in other societies, [that] it is preeminently reasonable to have fears about growing old.
>
> (Woodward, 1991: 23)

If Woodward is correct, what can be done to emancipate us from the fear of ageing and old age? How is it possible to foster positive attitudes towards the later part of life when the body finally wears out? At the present time the social construction of positive ageing both in everyday life and by the professionals attempts, as we have implied, to transform later life into an extended middle age terminating in a quick and painless exit: 'dying on time' as it is sometimes called. The associated practice is to transform the physical problems associated with the biological changes of later life (disability, confusion, social incompetence) first into social deviance – a process inevitably implying, if not explicitly requiring, moral discrimination and judgement – and second, as Gubrium (1986) shows in his analysis of the social construction of Alzheimer's Disease, to transform deviance in later life into evidence of clinical pathology. Behind this movement lies an often unspoken faith in the belief that if the decrements of later life are perceived as symptoms of a disease then it is not biological ageing that is to be feared but illness and the failure to combat ill health. Gubrium argues that one of the social advantages of the distinctive clinical category, Alzheimer's Disease, is that it can be utilised in two ways: (i) to establish and locate the cause of deviant behaviour in later life in clinical pathology – i.e. a deviant phenomenon endured by a minority (although the detected number of cases is apparently expanding); and (ii) to establish a social distance from normal physical ageing as experienced by the majority of older people in Western society. Although, as Gubrium shows, there are many problems associated with the accuracy of diagnosis, Alzheimer's Disease does have a demonstrable clinical existence and therefore acts as a scientifically sanctioned locus for the descriptive organisation of positive and negative ageing. If the ills of ageing can be attributed to physical pathology (biological deviation) then ageing itself is positively normal.

But there is a catch. Because it inevitably requires the social categorisation of bodies and behaviour, the message of 'positive ageing' is, as we have seen, a moral one. Writing, for example, in the magazine of the Association of Retired Persons (Summer 1993) in support of the current Government policy that expanding the costs of the NHS will have diminishing returns on the health of the nation, Dr David Weeks, a clinical psychologist, noted that 'One of the meaningful buzzwords now deployed in parts of the NHS is "empowerment". This is taken to be about helping people to take more positive action for themselves, thereby effecting improvements for themselves and others' (Weeks, 1993: 70). The broader message is one of the demedicalisation of normal ageing and its transformation into an arena for moral action. It is increasingly argued via the channels of health promotion that it is our duty to take precautions against the possible decrements of the future. Positive ageing has been validated in several unintentionally yet mutually supportive circles as the product of approved lifestyle choices and behaviours. The Summer 1993 issue of the *ARP 050 Reporter*, a companion broadsheet to the magazine *050*, contained three short paragraphs of comment on the BBC *Panorama* programme 'Dumping Grandma'. This programme focused on the problems facing some young people in caring for their parents and showed how Germany has passed legislation placing the cost of care firmly on the family. 'Will this happen in the UK?', the article enquired. 'It is our old age and infirmity, we are thinking about, let us face it now while we have the ability to organise insurances or pension schemes to cope with the situations that may arise' (Weeks, 1993: 2). The predominant solution is positive self-help usually with support of the services of approved commercial organisations and marketeers of age-related merchandise.

Yet another typical example of the contemporary imagery of positive ageing can be found on the cover of the Spring 1993 issue of *050*, which displayed a photograph of an exuberant middle-aged couple clinging lovingly together in a wild country garden. A central feature of the social construction of the imagery of positive ageing is the establishment of intimate nostalgic associations with sentimental visions of the (often 'olde English') countryside. Rustic imagery is thus not only a pervasive characteristic of images of successful retirement but also of bereavement as reflected in advertisements for prepaid funeral plans such as 'Golden Charter', illustrated in one widely circulating version by a photograph of an enchanting woodland scene where sunlight filters through autumnal leaves onto an older woman attending a pram and a small child on a leaf-strewn pathway.

PROVISIONAL CONCLUSION

Leo Miller observed that there are 'two kinds of problems of old age: those that older people actually have, and those that experts think they have' (Miller, 1987: 141). All of us working in the field of social gerontology, or who are concerned in any way about the care of older people, have a vested interest in creating a positive culture of ageing into old age. But it has been suggested in this chapter that if attention is paid to the sociology of social problems perspective a number of difficulties arise and that these difficulties can be traced to contradictions deeply embedded in Western culture and social organisation. One central contradiction, as Macintyre stressed in her paper of 1976, is between humanitarian and organisational interests. During the intervening period there have been no signs of a waning of this tension between the two interests; if anything the problem has become more acute, the currently favoured public solution reinforcing private efforts to marginalise the dependent old in the hope of normalising ageing and old age in a consumerist blur of rose-tinted 'normality'. Such action is essentially evasive and therefore ultimately repressive of the diversity in later life all gerontologists are exhorted to display and venerate. In his essay 'Becoming Deviant', Matza (1969) argued that there was an inherent conflict between efforts made towards the 'appreciation' of human diversity, that is a commitment to understanding phenomena as they occur in the natural social world, and the goal of 'ridding ourselves of the deviant phenomenon' (which he defined as a 'correctional' perspective). Whilst the correctional approach could at times be commendable it also stood in the way of 'empathy and understanding', sometimes making them 'impossible' (Matza, 1969: 15–17). At the same time he also detected an even greater problem arising out of the process of moral judgement inherent in correctionalism. Correctionalism was inevitably oversimplistic because it assumed that bad things (read here the physical decrements of old age) result from bad conditions, thus avoiding one of the central ironies of life, that good things also resulted in displeasing consequences.

For Matza the alternative perspective of 'appreciation' involved an understanding of the essential nature of 'overlap' and 'irony' (Matza, 1969: 68). 'Overlap' referred to the fact that in the real world of lived experience deviancy and normality were not necessarily sharply distinguishable one from the other. The margins between the two were often blurred. There was no 'dense barrier' (Matza, 1969: 69) separating deviance and normality and, as Gubrium (1986) later showed in his work on the social construction of Alzheimer's Disease, human beings have to work in association to create these boundaries and to ensure that they are maintained. 'Given the ironic tendency of naturalism', Matza wrote, 'bad things could result from highly treasured and revered aspects of social life, and good could be born of what was conventionally deemed evil' (Matza, 1969: 69). Irony therefore proposed a 'devious relation between virtue and vice' (1969: 77), a relation, it may be added, which is reflected all too frequently in ageing into old age.

In the context of the professional struggle to promote a positive interpretation of ageing into old age the picture that has emerged in this discussion is uncomfortably close to Cohen's 'likeliest future of social control' (Cohen, 1985: 232) – a future, as he envisaged it, of a 'decisive and deepening bifurcation: on the soft side there is indefinite inclusion, on the hard side, rigid exclusion' (1985: 232). Soft inclusive social control includes elements of positive ageing:

More domains of inner life will be penetrated in the same way as stages of the biological life span have been medicalised (life from birth to death as a series of risk periods, each calling for professional observation, check-ups, tutelage, supervision and intervention) or psychologised (by being turned into a series of growth periods, life crises, identity transitions or 'passages'). The cults of efficiency and happiness will offer themselves everywhere: posture, reflexes, orgasm, diet, breathing, dreams, relationships, psychic plumbing, child rearing

(Cohen, 1985: 232)

Yet, as other sociologists of ageing have observed, notably Norbert Elias in his characteristically unblinkered analysis of the plight of the old and the terminally sick in contemporary society (Elias, 1985), we must confront the social implications of the reality of biological ageing into old age if we are to establish genuinely positive attitudes towards old age and an aged population. The chief characteristic of prescriptions for positive ageing should be an ironic acceptance of the natural ending of one's life and therefore a critical response to the tendency in 'liberal capitalist culture' to display hostility towards physical decline and 'to regard health as a form of secular salvation' (Cole, 1992: 239).

Chapter 15

Health and lifestyle
A critical mess?
Notes on the dedifferentiation of health

Martin O'Brien

From the very outset, a symbolic expression for a verbally inexpressible state of affairs is created when we divide our inner existence into a central self and a surrounding array of contents.
Georg Simmel (1900) 'The Style of Life' in *The Philosophy of Money*
(1990 edition, pp. 472–3)

By 'life style' we refer to that orientation to self, others, and society, that each individual develops, that is, his value orientation.
Eli Ginzberg *et al.* (1966) *The Life Styles of Educated Women*, p. 145

Harold,' said Edith, 'I simply do not know anyone who has a lifestyle. What does it mean? It implies that everything you own was bought at exactly the same time, about five years ago, at the most.
Anita Brookner (1984) *Hotel du Lac*, pp. 26–7

INTRODUCTION

In this chapter I sketch out a sociological perspective on the development of key elements of health promotion ideology and practice. In particular, I consider the socio-political frameworks in which the new health movement has been able to intervene in a wider agenda for health. The discussion explores some of the origins of the extended concept of health upon which the movement relies and the relationships between this extension and more general socio-political changes of the last two decades. The purpose of the chapter is to situate health promotion in a sociological perspective on social and political change. To that end, the chapter is divided into four sections. In the first I offer some background comment on the concept of lifestyle. In the second, I discuss briefly the development of 'extended concepts' of health and, in particular, the expression of these in philosophies of 'wellbeing'. In the third section, I explore some of the sources from which such extended concepts derive. In the fourth section I address some key issues concerning the ways in which health promotion schemes are enmeshed in contradictory social, political and cultural influences. My argument is that lifestyle concepts, categories and projects are a vehicle of social differentiation: they serve to dislocate and disaggregate population sectors into targeted, bounded and discrete units. These 'units' are constructed through research and evaluation procedures, through marketing and administrative systems and through locally sensitive programmes and practical schemes. The consequence of the development of lifestyle-oriented practices has, however, led to the dedifferentiation of health in the context of wider social and political structures: they serve to 'open up' health to exogenous social, cultural, economic and political interests.

BACKGROUND

Social science has long been concerned with questions of lifestyle. Max Weber used the term when referring to social status categories, Georg Simmel's formal sociology exploited the idea in tackling the relationships between self and sociation, Alfred Adler employed 'life-style' as a label for personal uniqueness in a complex social world (Coreil and Levin, 1984). In each of these cases, the 'lifestyle' concept was intended to express both something essential and common – the process by which social identities and senses of self are constructed from available political, economic and cultural resources – and something ephemeral and specific – the inflection given to that process by the particular psycho-social characteristics of given individuals and groups. 'Lifestyle' implied 'choice' within a constrained context and the contexts were held to be more important than the choices. To address lifestyle was to address the social distribution of wealth, status and power and the impacts of these distributions on the ways that individuals and groups constituted their senses of self. To live a 'style' was both to respond to gross socio-economic divisions and to sustain the boundaries and barriers that comprised their social meanings. Today, 'lifestyle' has taken on an entirely different significance: far from depicting gross socio-cultural patterns through which divisions and distributions can be investigated, the term now functions as a means of overcoming those patterns and undermining the barriers that contain them.

However, in the sort of material irony that can only be generated by the intervention of powerful interests, this undermining and overcoming represents not a liberation from previously established inequalities and differences but an intensification and reactionary-political celebration of the social distinctions that modern society is endlessly capable of manufacturing. Today, lifestyle expresses nothing more than difference as such: it is the performance indicator *par excellence*, floating in a horizonless behavioural and attitudinal ocean, becoming ensnared in the nets of any institution fishing for targets to meet or niches to fill. Lifestyle, referring to nothing but itself, has emerged as a vehicle for differentiating a population, for breaking it apart, fragmenting its interests and distancing its members from forms of collective, social action. It is this fragmentation, breaking and distancing that lies at the heart of my discussion of the relationship between health and lifestyle, a relationship I see as being *critical* in the sense of embodying a moment of political change from which there is no turning back: lifestyle projects in health promotion programmes are partners of more deeply embedded social and political processes affecting contemporary social life. The association between 'health' and 'lifestyle' is fundamentally a political achievement, supported by an institutionalised consumerism, validated by a liberal political ideology and nurtured by a technocratic professionalism increasingly oriented towards problem solving approaches to health and social life. If, at the end of the 1970s, everyday life had become increasingly medicalised (Crawford, 1980), by the end of the 1980s, health had become increasingly personalised, fragmented and 'styled' in a repoliticisation of health knowledge and practice.[1]

FROM HEALTH TO WELLBEING

Health workers, health policy makers, health analysts and health service users are increasingly being urged to 'extend' their understandings of health, its causes, dimensions and treatments. These calls can be found in health philosophy, in the health curriculum, in policy statements, in academic debate about the distribution and consequences of health and disease patterns, and in codes of professional practice (see, *inter alia*, World Health Organisation (1984), Mahler (1986), Novak (1988), Catford and Parish (1989), Open University (1992–3)). The extension is intended to introduce: a reconceptualisation of health; a new way of seeing health; a new way of coming to know what health is; and a widening of the meaning of health from an absence of disease or physical functioning to include social issues, such as transport, work, housing, sexuality and the politics of risk and choice as well as behavioural and attitudinal factors. The extended concept places health at the intersection of key life experiences and conditions and implies a multidimensional agenda for health policy and practice.

Variations on this wider perspective have been taken up in different fields of health delivery and are applied in area-specific projects (in the different branches of nursing and medicine, in District Health Authorities, hospitals and Local Authority Environmental Health Departments, at work, in schools, in general practice and so on). Although many such projects express common objectives (notably, reductions in heart and lung diseases and cancers) they are in important ways parallel rather than unified enterprises. They are funded from different sources (from the market, industry and charity as well as general taxation disbursed by innumerable different authorities), have different aims and goals (such as a healthy workforce, stress reduction, dietary change, communicating health information), are controlled by different institutional and individual actors (for example, general practitioners, health promotion officers, local authorities and personnel departments) and adopt different operational targets (such as reductions in absenteeism, increased take-up of services or meeting screening targets and the provision of healthy diets). Populations are defined according to the needs of the project rather than the agenda of the members themselves.

On the one hand, the diversity and ubiquity of these strategies suggests a lively and committed pattern of interventions into the causes and consequences of ill-health and the definition and application of resources for health. On the other, they raise questions about the political framework in which lifestyle and wellness interventions are constructed. This becomes clear when the goals and purposes of the diversity are openly stated – rather than remaining as subterranean themes in projects targeted at specific health conditions. A clear and concise statement of the value of a wider health agenda is provided in the Open University's *Health and Wellbeing* (1992–3) course – a practitioner-centred training package designed to educate health workers into new ways of thinking and working for wellness. Here, the diversity of research, projects and interventions is applauded because it is:

> essential that health remains an arena of open debate and dialogue so that policies can continue to be modified and changed and new social movements and cultural influences can be encompassed in the health agenda of the future.
>
> (Open University, 1992–3, Workbook 3: 100)

These types of normative statements are legion across all the social and political sciences. The desire to incorporate and assimilate multiple voices into institutional and professional practice is as common in the critical literature today as were questions of class in the 1970s. What is less common in the new health literature is the self-critical appraisal of that goal and the means to its achievement. Key questions remain to be posed of health promotion whilst its radical vision remains in sight. What, for example, are the consequences of 'opening' the arena of health, of widening the remit of health so that its (professional) representatives can discourse on subjects as diverse as work, transport and lifestyle? Who gains and who loses from such an 'opening' and precisely what form of 'opening' are we talking about? From where has this extended concept of 'health-as-wellbeing' derived and what sort of social and political change is represented by the development of a system in which a much wider range of beliefs, statuses and knowledges becomes the object of health surveillance and intervention? If we encourage the assimilation of social movements and cultural influences into the health agenda, are we effectively undermining cultural autonomy and deflecting social protest into technologies and systems for their management and administration rather than liberating multiple voices from the oppressive silence that traditional medical histories seemingly impose on them? It is in questions like these that the distinction between practitioner perspectives and sociological perspectives is most obvious. Gains and losses, assimilations and surveillance, are central political dimensions of health promotion practice and organisation, key features of what health promotion represents as a social phenomenon. In order to understand the significance of new health perspectives and programmes sociologically therefore, it is necessary that these are placed in a wider social and political context, one that makes connections between the types of perspective and programme on offer and key changes in the material and ideological conditions surrounding them.

It is in this sense that the extended conceptualisation of health can be said to represent a critical moment in the development of new health programmes because it achieves, and is itself an element of, wider social changes. The extension of health into the area of wellbeing can be understood as a process of *dedifferentiation* (or 'opening up') of health in the context of everyday life: a dedifferentiation in which goals, values, statuses, rights and duties have coalesced around new socio-political rationalities. These rationalities, which I discuss in the following sections of this chapter, have served to transform health from a state or condition to be achieved and valued into a systemic surveillance process: continual – voluntary and involuntary – monitoring now stands at the pinnacle of healthy practice; innumerable fine-tunings applied to behaviour patterns, nutritional balances, relaxation techniques and even modes of thought and belief line the route that defines how healthy lives are conducted. This route, in keeping with contemporary theories of modern society,[2] can be thought of as a motorway travelling from birth to death. Like motorways in Britain, the road is lined with expensive service stations. Those who have sufficient resources can afford, when they choose, to purchase a three course meal at the healthy options food counter; those travelling on a much tighter budget must make do with coffee and cheap pastries. So it is with contemporary health practice: the individually over-resourced are offered opportunities to achieve integration and balance between home, leisure, work, diet, sense of self and all the other 'risk factors' that define modern life; the individually under-resourced must prioritise according to complex need-calculations involving self and others and these calculations call for sacrifices and structured choices deriving precisely from the constraints imposed by home, work, diet, leisure and sense of self.

Socially organising these two poles of access is a system of power-knowledge: one in which populations are assimilated into and distributed around a health sector that is simultaneously expanding and contracting, a process fuelled by the integration of health and wellness. The sector's expansion comprises an extended *remit over* life – from genetic manipulation to euthanasia via holistic therapies and workforce screening. Its contraction is observed in a reduced *obligation to* life – health is constructed as a series of encounters with risk factors in diet and behaviour, at work and play, in public and private networks, factors that can be monitored and correlated, channelled and controlled, prioritised and targeted. Health – as absence of disease, functional or adaptive capacity or physical constitution – is no longer enough. Today's travellers on the road to corporal salvation are urged also to acquire, to produce and to value 'wellbeing', such that assimilation into health today is assimilation into a network of structured choices circulating in a chaotic marketplace of stylistic options. The extended concept of health-as-wellbeing represents a biographical project, requiring knowledge of social, psychological, political and economic processes. It is multifactorial, multisectoral and multidimensional; a probabilistic patterning of encounters and adaptations in everyday life.

This contradiction – of simultaneous expansion and contraction – raises questions about the medicalisation thesis: the increasing encroachment of the profession and power of medicine into larger and larger fractions of the public and private spheres (Illich, 1976; Ehrenreich, 1978; Crawford, 1980). The medicalisation thesis has been a powerful tool for understanding key social changes and the roles of powerful professions in achieving change. Yet it is also clear that the encroachment is neither simple nor unidirectional. Responsibility for and obligation to health shift, in the focus on wellbeing, between health workers and patients, families, communities, employers, educators and the voluntary and charitable sectors. The extended concept of health does not in any simple sense represent increasing power for medical professionals. For such a shift requires at least that the characteristics of these actors and the contours of these institutions are an integrated component of health delivery. It requires that sociological, political, economic and cultural rationalities – as well as the rationalities of technological medicine – underpin health philosophies, priorities and practices. The expanded concept of health that I am describing is synthetic, created by a particular dedifferentiation of health and social life. It is the epistemological outcome of an assimilation of health into key political rationalities whose origins, development and control lie outside medical discourse. This assimilation is nowhere more apparent than in the intersection of health and lifestyles.

THE POLITICS OF LIFESTYLE

In 1981, Sobel opened his book on *Lifestyle and Social Structure*, with the prediction that 'If the 1970s are an indication of things to come, the word lifestyle, will soon include everything and mean nothing, all at the same time' (Sobel, 1981: 1). The prediction was accurate; there is no longer anything that does not belong to the sphere of 'lifestyle' and there is no meaning sufficiently flexible to connect the diverse referents to which the concept applies.[3] Yet the explosion in contents and referents has occurred neither by chance nor strictly by design. It can be traced to three discrete sources of ignition that entered public space in the 1960s and 1970s and began to merge together from the middle of the 1980s onwards.

One source can be located in political-economic shifts from the 1960s that currently form the basis of the Post-Fordism debate (Murray, 1989) and is best articulated in new systems of product marketing. These marketing philosophies began to eschew gross, *objective* consumption sectors based on socio-economic position (or class) in favour of *subjective* market segments based on specific behavioural and attitudinal characteristics (Willis, 1990). From the 1970s onwards, such marketing strategies became increasingly sophisticated. Together with growing social science interest in consumption this segmentation served to undermine traditional class-based accounts of social and political cultures (Douglas and Isherwood, 1979; Featherstone, 1987). In finer and finer detail social scientists, advertisers and market researchers have differentiated consumption behaviours into 'lifestyle' categories and in so doing have assisted the development of increasingly specific frameworks for both product distribution and political expression.

For example, Townsend and Riche (1987) produced a seven-segment measure of lifestyles in married households (Honeymooners, Just-a-couples, New-parents, Young Families, Full Nesters, Crowded Nesters, and Empty Nesters); Schwarz (1988) examined the buying patterns of consumers in the USA and developed a four-segment lifestyle typology to account for their purchasing behaviour (Harried, Traditional, Financially Restricted and Working Singles); Exter (1987) took up work by Peter Earl to describe 'lifestyle economics' in terms of a three-segment model of how consumers cope with uncertainty (Enterprising Consumers, Inquisitive Consumers, and Evolving Consumers). Gattas *et al.* (1986) sought to promote a leisure research agenda based on the concept of lifestyle. Arguing that 'lifestyle' has thus far achieved no operational definition they proposed a 'reconceptualisation' based on the relationship between time structures of individuals and groups and consumption patterns. Khakhulina (1984) had a similar (operationalisation) goal in mind but produced a fourfold conceptual scheme to account for the interrelation between living standard and lifestyle (comprising indicators of consumption, the structure of needs, citizens, activities and the time allotted to these). Bertaux (1983) argued that everyday life can only be analysed with reference to specific lifestyle frameworks considered as modes of reproduction and proposed a seven-segment typology based on the relationships between needs and available resources (Destitution, Poverty, Need, Sufficiency, Affluence, Wealth and Power). Davis and French (1989) targeted 'the aged', Lastovicka and Joachminsthaler (1988) targeted 'pet-owners', Donohew *et al.* (1987) targeted 'media-users' whilst Shama (1988) merged 'materialist' and 'postmaterialist' value frameworks in unpacking the behaviour of 'voluntary simplicity consumers' (O'Brien, 1992). Lifestyle marketing in new public health schemes adopts the same techniques and methods for disaggregating the social, cultural and economic characteristics of its service users (Lefebvre and *et al.*, 1988).

The sample of material discussed above is itself a tiny proportion of the great variety of concepts and frameworks that have emerged across the last two decades. It is important to recognise how difficult it is at first to make any connections between these different schemas, segments, sections and fractions of collective life; the obscurity of the categories themselves is deepened by the disunity that they represent taken together. The relationship between 'Empty-nesters', the 'Destitute' or the 'structure of needs', and so on, is both ambiguous – in the sense that it is not clear that the researchers have even begun from the same conception of the human actor's experiences, needs and goals – and ambivalent – in the sense that what links together the different schema is precisely that they are fragments, that they combine and recombine differences as the core of the analysis. Each schema draws differently on economic and social, psychological and cultural variables and each is differently productive: they serve the ends of social science in establishing new research and theoretical agenda, the ends of political and policing authorities in identifying socio-economic or demographic concentrations of deviance,[4] the ends of capitalist enterprise by enabling the realisation of exchange value in the market, the ends of professions in demarcating client and, today, customer groups. They represent, in theory and in practice, a differentiation of collective life. In this sense the lifestyle movement appears as a modern technology: a means of dividing life experience into discrete and autonomous segments and, like Foucault's (1977) disciplined inmates, subjecting each segment to experimentation and normalisation in everything from product design through advertising strategies to sociological research and individual health.

Yet, these principles for associating, aggregating and organising populations – in networks and not hierarchies, around value-sets and not positional groups, in terms of specific goals and not generalised allegiances – were and are also characteristic of the second source for lifestyle concepts: counter-cultural movements.[5] Of special significance here are the ecology movements, which generated sustained critiques of overconsumption, waste and materialism. Schumacher's (1974) *Small is Beautiful*, Roszak's (1981) *Person/Planet*, and Porritt's (1990) *Seeing Green* articulate well this movement in lifestyle politics. Stressing individual responsibility and self-reliance, the integrated totality of the material, the mental and the spiritual, the counter-cultures offered alternative ideologies of the present and visions of the future rooted in a transformation of environmental ethics and a repersonalisation of political choices. Ideologically, they served to break down existing boundaries between production and consumption, work and home, public and private and to promote new cultural identities based on shared experiences, goals and values. Counterculture groups challenged politically the dissection of personal experience and collective action. Forging connections between consumption and ecological damage, patriarchy and sexual oppression, the body and social regulation involved linking together practices and experiences that were previously socially and culturally exclusive, bounded and differentiated.

Consciousness-raising groups, peace networks and movements for sexual liberation shared informalised modes of association, non-hierarchical organisation and issue-specific campaigning strategies. Many of these orientations formed the basis of challenges to public institutions through the self-help movement including the women's health movement, which aimed to wrest control over women's bodies from the male professional structures and hierarchies associated with medicine (Rich, 1977; Leeson and Gray, 1978; Orr, 1988). These critiques extend well beyond the health sector itself to challenge and overturn patriarchal concepts of citizenship and social participation (Lister, 1990; Walby, 1994).

The political reorientation introduced by counter-culture pressure is a key dimension of new health ideologies. The *Ottawa Charter for Health Promotion* (WHO, 1986a) emphasised strengthening community action, enabling personal development and creating supportive environments as well as stressing the importance of public policy and official health organisations. The focus on community networks and local action (for example Ashton, 1988), on the need to validate the everyday health work of different local actors (Bryant, 1988) and on the reconstruction of public services parallels the 'new group politics' (Beer, 1982) of contemporary social movements. This is because, like the ecology, peace, disabled rights and anti-racist movements, health work now involves the generation of alliances across consumer–producer, local–global and public–private divisions.

In important respects, then, traces of counter-cultural themes pervade new health philosophies. The relationship between the individual and the social and, more rarely, the personal and the political, is represented as a combination of particular choices and general constraints (of education, custom and class, for example) and it is this combination that drives forward the practical and organisational assimilation of health into multiple institutional sites. In the practice of operating cross-sectoral delivery, and in reconciling the different interests and values contained within the sectors, a common political territory has been demarcated that inserts individual behaviours, attitudes, resources and roles (the objects of health promotion practice) into locally styled projects. Lifestyle has come to represent a vehicle that can carry competing ideologies, disciplinary techniques, and economic and social priorities: a neutralised political space in which individualised 'wellness' behaviour can be measured and matched with institutionally controlled resources.

A third source for the expansion of lifestyle referents is tied to the critique of modernisation and, in its wake, the critique of modernity and the rigid systems of organisation characteristic of modern society. The critique of modernisation was part of a political readjustment of social development policies across the 1970s. These include the Community Development projects in India, Africa and South America – parallelled in the Community Development Programmes in British cities from the late 1960s to the late 1970s (Loney, 1983) – together with the Club of Rome's *Limits to Growth*, and the World Health Organisation's (1978) Alma Ata declaration. These programmes and policies stressed autonomy, self-determination, decentralisation, equity, participation and a reorganisation of public institutions and services in order to generate appropriate social development programmes, tailored to the socio-cultural characteristics of particular populations and operating according to locally specific priorities and needs. Bolstered by experiences in developing countries (Morley *et al.*, 1987) this political shift established the recognition of diversity and difference as key dimensions in the restructuring of health and welfare systems. As the focus of health philosophy extended into new cultural questions, the contours and the practice of everyday life became critical tools in the redefinition and redistribution of health resources.

The critique of modern health systems and the analytical and political response to it has been contradictory, a fact that can be seen in the proposals of one of the major players in the health promotion movement – the World Health Organisation (WHO). The WHO has acted as a catalyst for shifts in the makeup of regional health policies in every continent of the globe. Stressing the central importance of family, neighbourhood, school, work and other 'local' frameworks of action the WHO has been keen to connect health with social and economic variables operating in the immediate contexts of people's everyday choices. The WHO has pressured national and regional health organisations to adopt multidisciplinary and multisectoral working patterns in order to integrate the details of people's ways of living into organisational philosophies and practices.

Supporting the integration is a research programme designed to generate complex, multidimensional information on personal, social and economic variables. This is because 'very little is known' about the interactions between beliefs, lifestyles and health behaviour with the consequence that

> Basic research on the determinants of healthy or unhealthy lifestyles will have to be expanded to deal with such questions as how known determinants such as social integration actually perform their mediating and health-producing or health-protecting roles.
>
> (WHO, 1986b: 121)

The research will furnish health workers with knowledge about the ways that families, communities and workplaces function in maintaining or undermining health. Contradictorily, the WHO acknowledges that a variety of personal and social relations have been objectified in traditional medical programmes – family relations, child development and types of 'deviance' (WHO, 1986b: 122) – but still proposes that this objectification in the name of health should be extended. The objectification takes the form of a factorisation and a reconstruction: multiple 'risk' variables are plotted and evaluated by professional researchers and are recombined by local operatives in a bewildering variety of campaigns (healthy diets, AIDS awareness, seat belt use, stress reduction and so on). Cultural priorities, social networks, community organisations and economic resources serve both to establish the boundaries of local health systems and to control and validate specific health programmes. The consequence is a shift in the nature and hierarchy of what is objectified in the organisation of health systems. Not only specific categories of deviance, particular stages of child development and distinctive patterns of family relationship, but the whole patterned range of activity, the entirety of locally available types of social and economic organisation and the dominant beliefs, values and attitudes of people living their everyday lives are legitimate targets for the new public health.

LIFESTYLES AND HEALTH PROMOTION

The association between health and lifestyle represents a *mess* because the intersection of these three sources – deriving from movements in civil society, the economy and politics – has created a confusion of competing interests which today is amalgamated in the concept and practice of health promotion. On the one hand, the health promotion movement represents an almost ideal discursive system – able to draw on value sources emphasising autonomy and empowerment and generating frameworks for understanding a democratised health, technical sources emphasising procedures for targeting relevant groups and channelling behaviours via the manipulation of values, and political sources generating policies for the focused delivery of health in locally discrete and 'lifestyle sensitive' programmes. On the other hand, health promotion represents a movement intrinsically in tension with itself, attempting to reconcile the requirements of different actors. As the intersection of these multiple sources of influence the health promotion movement has been a key player in the normalisation of lifestyle categories as legitimate targets, values and criteria for health. The contradictory goals, interests and practices of the movement are reconnected in a new form of institutionalised delivery that subjects health to the forces of competing social, cultural, political and economic organisations. In this sense, it is not everyday life that has been colonised in the name of health, but health that has been colonised in the name of 'lifestyle'.

The diversity of the health projects aimed at widening the concept and remit of health through lifestyle manipulation matches the diversity of social science and marketing projects aimed at unpacking life style characteristics. They include attention to the health of menopausal women (McLennan, 1993), working-class mothers (Pill *et al.*, 1993), adolescents (Joliff *et al.*, 1992), gays and lesbians (Dankmeijer, 1993), health at work (Webb and Schilling, 1988), dietary practices (Holm, 1993), heart disease (Blackburn *et al.*, 1984; Puska *et al.*, 1985; Ornish *et al.*, 1990), psychiatric morbidity (Anderson *et al.*, 1993), the homeless and socially marginal (Schnabel, 1992), the status of patients (Stott and Pill, 1990; Kelly, 1992), among many others, as well as referring solely to the efficacy of health-promoting lifestyles in general (Gillis, 1993).

Under the analytic banner of lifestyle and the ideological goal of well-being, delivering health services consists in the effort to reconcile a plethora of social, personal, political, economic and environmental variables. These variables are profiled (using the techniques of anthropology, organisational development and community psychology (WHO, 1986b: 121) among others) within populations as 'risk factors'. Such profiles map social, behavioural and health characteristics of both 'communities' (for example, Winchester Health Promotion Department (1989), Milton Keynes Health Authority (1987) and Oxford RHA (1987)) and individuals (for example, Hunt *et al.* (1985) and Pembrokeshire HA (1988)). To achieve individual health is to steer a route through risks that cannot be avoided; to deliver health is to counter the risk effect of personal, social, environmental and cultural hazards. The issue of risk and health is becoming an increasingly significant element of both health research and philosophy (see, for example, Scott *et al.*, 1992). The recent (USA) litigation against secondary smoking effects, the confused (UK) debate over repetitive strain injury, the correlation between chest disease and proximity to traffic and fears over pesticides and food additives point to the extremes of a shift in responsibility for health risks. In various combinations, working conditions, food production systems, cultural practices, ecological damage and housing choices are weighed against individual needs and expectations. At the same time, businesses, workers' associations, schools and community organisations take over key roles in monitoring, evaluating and countering those same 'health risks'. Providing healthy options in the canteen, segregating smokers and non-smokers, conducting drink-awareness campaigns, encouraging exercise, reorganising workplaces, forming self-help groups (or Look After Yourself groups, in the aptly named scheme sponsored by the Health Education Authority), developing worker welfare policies and distributing health education everywhere from the surgery to the local carnival through posters, leaflets, speeches and videos forge multiple lines of administration and influence over life choices made by people in their everyday social, cultural, political and economic contexts. Conrad and Walsh (1992), for example, investigating trends in North American industry, suggest that the boundary between private and public is being blurred in the name of workplace health. Employee assistance programmes, drug screening and wellness schemes target dimensions of workers' lifestyles both inside and outside the workplace. Being 'well', in the terms of these programmes – i.e. in financial, emotional, social and physical terms – amounts to a corporate ethic that extends beyond the domain of work into domestic contexts and leisure activities.

The incorporation of lifestyle factors into systems for delivering health thus comprises a change in the ways that population groups encounter 'health care' and, indeed, into the forms that providing for health takes. On the one hand, 'lifestyles' are commodified frameworks that can be sold (Rice, 1988) through social marketing techniques (Manos, 1985; Lefebvre et al., 1988). Here, health is constructed as a commodity that can be sold to segmented consumer groups in order to enhance their 'wellbeing'. Health promotion programmes are designed to persuade individuals to 'purchase' or 'adopt' different types of lifestyle, depending upon their degree of consumer power – including both their financial capacity to acquire particular goods and services and also their status as 'champion' or potentially powerful exemplar of particular lifestyle characteristics (Catford and Parish, 1989). On the other hand, where simple (or sophisticated) persuasion techniques fail, a surveillance apparatus geared towards evaluating the development of the range of personal, social and cultural variables waits in the wings. Being 'not-ill' is only one part of the array of assessments, interventions, measurements and campaigns designed to ensure the development of personal wellness. Simultaneously, being 'not-well' is in no measure simply the responsibility of or under the authority of a medically oriented health system rooted in technological or allopathic treatments. A socio-cultural rationality intervenes alongside rationalities of commodification and cure. By encapsulating the multiple dimensions of everyday life in the concept of lifestyle, the promotion of wellness encourages the establishment of new institutional alliances between economic, cultural and social interests. The individual and collective assimilation into 'wellness' is thus itself an assimilation into a political framework that is crossed by contradictory rationalities, targets and policies.

Health is no longer a matter of medicine, bodily function, or even spaces of disease distribution (Armstrong, 1983). Contemporary health is a fusion of social, economic and cultural styles and contexts. Values, behaviours and emotional sets, transport choices, working conditions and educational provision are 'resources' for health that can be channelled and targeted, manipulated and 'corrected'. This is a process in continual flux, subjected to the rationalities and structures of institutions as diverse as employers, community groups, political organisations and welfare services as well as those traditionally associated with the health sector. It is in this sense that health has been dedifferentiated into everyday life; for, now, health is derived from its social, economic and cultural dimensions in an absolute and critical reversal of medicine's relation to the social body. Where, for medical science, the body of the patient acted as the prime source and object of health, for health promoters the wellness of individuals is a product of their lifestyle. Far from a medicalisation of 'health', medicine is relegated to one structure among others from which a particular biographical 'wellbeing' is socially constructed.

CONCLUDING COMMENTS

The health promotion movement today is the product of many forces, both endogenous and exogenous to the health system. These forces are simultaneously political, economic, social and cultural, and this intersection creates a confusing and contradictory social programme of health maintenance. Within an ideology of holistic wellness the contradictions appear as ambiguous and ambivalent constructions of lifestyle characteristics in new networks of knowledge, action and resources. These networks both challenge and maintain divisions between the public and the private, home and work, the individual and the social in the actual delivery of health services. The intersection of the disparate interests of economic, social and political actors has resulted in a 'critical mess' through which 'health' has been dispersed into non-medical surveillance and maintenance systems that target behaviours and beliefs, norms and mores and blur the boundaries between public and private, individual and social life in the name of 'wellness'. This extended concept of health is a consequence of the socio-political development of health promotion and not a vision that unites its multidimensional project.

NOTES

1 This ideological and practical twist to the tale of health services development is a stronger indication of the emergence of a life politics than any 'Utopian realist' social movement (Giddens, 1990); but it is a life politics that is imposed in an institutional reconstruction of health resources rather than one that reflexively and unproblematically brings new moral issues to the public agenda.
2 Giddens (1990) describes the experience of modern society as like riding a juggernaut. I am simply extending the metaphor to acknowledge that juggernauts need fuel and their drivers need nourishment.
3 Including Sobel's own as 'a distinctive, hence recognizable, mode of living' (Sobel, 1981: 19).
4 Whether defined in terms of poverty, health or criminality.
5 It is interesting to note that the *Humanities Index* changed its system of entries in the mid-1980s, replacing the category 'counter-culture' with 'lifestyle'.

Chapter 16

Consumption and health in the 'epidemiological' clinic of late modern medicine

Robin Bunton and Roger Burrows

INTRODUCTION

This chapter draws upon work from the sociology of consumption and the sociology of health and illness in order to explore the relationship between health promotion and 'health-related' consumer culture. It argues that health promotion has emerged within contemporary consumer culture and is centrally concerned with influencing patterns of consumer choice. Under contemporary consumer culture consumption preferences are determined by a wide range of social factors that interact in complex ways with the discourse of health promotion. The chapter concludes that health promotion would benefit greatly by coming to terms with cultural aspects of the interaction between consumption, risk and health, and, conversely, shifting away from its current emphasis upon individual and psychological aspects of health-related behaviour (Bunton *et al.*, 1991).

HEALTH PROMOTION AS LATE MODERN MEDICINE

Health promotion self-consciously attempts to define itself as a new approach to health care. It deliberately distances itself from more traditional hospital-centred curative medicine and attempts to forge a reconceptualisation of health, no longer defined in contradistinction to illness, but redefined positively as akin to wellbeing. This is primarily articulated in terms of the promotion of lifestyles supposedly conducive to health as well as various attempts to minimise preventable conditions. At the risk of some simplification, health promotion can perhaps best be viewed in relation to a number of polarities between two ideal types of 'old' and 'new' systems of health care, the 'old' system being paradigmatic of modernism, and the 'new' of late modernism.[1] We have attempted to represent this in Figure 16.1.

Within this framework, medicine of the modern period is characterised as: curative; institutionally based; built upon the expertise of a narrow group of professionals; and requiring a heavy investment of resources directed towards relatively passive individuals. By contrast, late modern public health, of which health promotion is a central feature, is characterised as: preventative; non-institutional; multisectoral; multidisciplinary; not necessarily requiring the heavy utilisation of resources; and conducted only with the active participation of groups and social networks. Under this description health promotion and the new public health represent new forms of social mediation in relation to health and illness. Whilst the bio-medical model relies upon focused interactions between professionals and patients within a clinical setting, the new public health widens the relevant points of social contact into myriad different sites, locations and social interactions oriented towards the social body.

'Old' bio-medical health care	'New' public health care
Curative	Preventative
Institutional	Non-institutional
Specialist	Non-specialist
High cost	Low cost
Individual focused	Group focused
Non-participative	Participative
Clinics	Epidemiology
Dangerousness	Risk
Modern	Late modern

Figure 16.1 Some contrasts between 'old' and 'new' health care systems

THE CHANGING SICK ROLE AND THE EMERGENCE OF THE 'EPIDEMIOLOGICAL' CLINIC

Although the subject of extensive criticism (Gerhardt, 1987), the Parsonian concept of the sick role (Parsons, 1951; 1958; 1975) provides a familiar heuristic device that can be used to explore some aspects of this shift towards a late modern system of health care. In Parsons' classic account of modern medicine the status of the sick actor was essentially accounted for by his or her separation from everyday activities and other people in a cycle of insulation and, upon regaining health, subsequent reintegration into the social system. Sickness ascription relieved the actor from fulfilling normal duties at work, in the family and elsewhere and (in welfare states) ensured some income and support whilst occupying this status. Under this description the sick are absolved from responsibility for the duration of their temporary incapacity. In return for this status they are obliged to attempt to get better and also to seek expert assistance and comply with any recommended treatment regime to this end. The sick role under modernism thus brings people into contact with *specific* therapeutic agencies and places them in a position of dependency in relation to those who are not sick. Thus, sickness is a state that is largely individualised and involves recovery in private or domestic sites usually clearly demarcated from work, leisure and other public spheres.

Contrast this with the sick role implied by the late modern regime with its emphasis on health promotion. Whilst the rights and duties of the sick may still be applied to a number of *episodic* states of sickness these are now extensively augmented by a number of other *continuous* professional interventions affecting not just the sick person and her or his immediate associates, but also the general 'healthy' population as well. The contemporary citizen is increasingly attributed with responsibilities to ceaselessly maintain and improve her or his own health by using a whole range of measures. To do this she or he is increasingly expected to take note of and act upon the recommendations of a whole range of 'experts' and 'advisers' located in a range of *diffuse* institutional and cultural sites. Health promotion activities take place in a great many locations, many of which are outside the traditional institutional domains associated with the sick role: we experience them on TV and radio in our homes; we experience them at the workplace in employee assistance programmes; we are presented with literature and other promotions in our pubs, clubs, sports centres, supermarkets and shopping malls; and we may even find literature arriving with our pay cheques to remind us of sensible drinking levels. There is now virtually no site that is left unexplored.

The duties that health promotion invokes have thus been added to those of the sick role. However, they are also duties that extend well beyond this domain in that they have also begun to constitute important new late modern social roles for everyone: *health* roles. These changes may be understood as part of a wider move towards greater *reflexivity* in late modern subjectivity (Giddens, 1991) – the idea that more and more aspects of social life can be subject to strategic transformation and modification on the basis of new knowledge and the capacity to discursively interpret conduct. We are thus concerned with the development of a new form of governance, one that has moved well beyond the walls of the hospital and involves not just the physician and the patient, but a whole range of agencies dispersed throughout society requiring of the individual an extension of their concerns 'with body boundaries' and 'individual psychology' to 'lifestyle' more generally (Armstrong, 1993b: 405).

Castel (1991) provides a useful way of conceptualising this transformation by suggesting that we are entering a new paradigm of health care (Nettleton, 1995). He claims that we are moving from a health care system premised upon 'dangerousness' to one based upon 'risk'. Hitherto, he argues, health professionals have tended to err on the side of caution to prevent any manifestation of disease and, consequently, the illnesses possessed by patients have been treated as being potentially dangerous. However, in the contemporary period the target of medical care is, he argues, shifting from the *symptoms* of concrete individuals to their *charac-*

teristics, which the discourses of health promotion and prevention have constituted as risk factors. For Castel the 'clinic of the subject' is being replaced by an ' "epidemiological" clinic, a system of multifarious but exactly localized expertise which supplants the old doctor–patient relation. This certainly does not mean the end of the doctor, but it does definitely mark a profound transformation in medical practice' (Castel, 1991: 282).

Thus, he suggests, we are witnessing the advent of a new mode of surveillance, aided by technological advances, which make the calculus and probabilities of 'systematic pre-detection' more and more sophisticated. Populations are thereby increasingly being managed on the basis of their profiles in relation to factors such as their age, social class, occupation, gender, relationships, locality, lifestyle and consumption. It is factors such as these, and their particular configurations, that form the basis of risk. This transformation is, of course, part of a wider shift in the operations of the technologies of power under late modernism; it represents another instance of the displacement of sovereign power by disciplinary power over the body (Nettleton and Burrows, 1994).

This shift is already evident in much of the contemporary health care system in the growth of needs assessments based on epidemiological and survey data. Further, strategies are being devised to improve collective health status rather than that of individuals. These strategies identify targets in the form of the collective reduction of risk factors and the development of a network of effective health care and social services. Health promotion practioners' conceptions of their occupational role also clearly concur with this image of the 'at a distance' management of people. Work under the rubric of contemporary health promotion and new public health thus falls firmly within these new patterns of health and social care: it is work directed at populations, those that are well, at risk or experiencing ill-health of some kind; it draws on increasingly more systematic surveillance and the monitoring of behaviour in increasing detail; and it attempts to engineer intervention regimes that take place in highly dispersed settings, managed and coordinated by a wide range of agents. Whilst the health promotion sites of the 'epidemiological' clinic are primarily thought of as being in the 'community', the social and physical space occupied by this category is altogether more diffuse under late modernism. It is an increasingly commodified space, at its most dense at the sites of consumption.

HEALTH PROMOTION, CONSUMPTION AND SELF-IDENTITY

Consumption sites form a crucial aspect of health promotion discourses for three reasons. First, communities, for so long the uncritical focus of much health promotion discourse, are 'not what they used to be'. The often idealised 'community' is, under late modernism, increasingly immersed and experienced from within consumer culture. Whilst we may not agree with Baudrillard's exaggerated claim that the 'social' is disappearing we can acknowledge that routine daily life in 'communities' is becoming increasingly mediated by consumption and new technological forms (Baudrillard, 1981; Rheingold, 1994). Thus, in orienting towards the community, health promotion now inevitably enters ever more deeply into the domain of consumer culture.

Second, the focus and methods of health promotion are intimately implicated in marketing. Illness prevention in public health has been seen as the outcome of the interaction of key variables: potentially harmful agents (micro-organisms, food, drugs, etc.), the host (the human form), and the environment (the spaces in which the former variables interact). It is significant that health promotion rhetoric has rearticulated these into products, people and places (WHO, 1988a). The regulation of harmful products advocated by public policy initiatives recognises the conflict of interest between consumers and producers – policy on tobacco production and marketing being a case in point. Whilst the wider politics of health issues are identified in this rhetoric, much of current practice in health promotion relies on marketing campaigns and on the individualising of consumption issues. Social marketing 'theory', developed under the auspices of health promotion, attempts to develop a methodology and techniques to market social change in the name of health (Lefebvre, 1992), placing health promotion within a more general promotional culture (Bunton, 1991; Wernick, 1991). Such an approach condenses product regulation to the level of an individual calculus of consumption. The propensity towards various forms of ill health is reformulated as a function of the supposed 'health-giving' or 'sick-making' properties of various commodities and/or activities, almost all of which are now firmly located in the symbolic domain of consumer culture – smoking, drinking, sport and exercise, diet and so on. Health is idealised as self-governed lifestyle choice. Health promotion and the new public health attempt to cultivate consumption preferences driven by the reflexive calculation, monitoring and recalibration of commodity inputs in the pursuit of health. However, for many social groups the health consumption calculus promulgated by the social marketing of health promotion is fettered by other powerful cultural forces also at play at the same sites of consumption (cigarette and alcohol advertising for example). Below, by way of an example, we consider this play of cultural forces in the context of an analysis of contemporary patterns of drug use.

Third, under late modernism the dominant culture is one in which health, self-identity and consumption are increasingly entwined. The aggregate effects of this cultural affinity often all but drown out any independent efficacy that health promotion discourses *per se* may possess. The growth in 'health-related' goods and services might be explicable in terms of a logic of capitalism in which markets have to be constantly opened up for new commodities. From this perspective, public concerns with health as wellbeing are welcomed and encouraged by capital in order to buttress the sale of commodities not just to the sick but also to the well. Although this economic imperative is undoubtedly important, a deeper and more important cultural dynamic is also at play here. Health promotion is symptomatic of wider cultural change involving the fabrication of more reflexive late modern self-identities. This in turn demands of the self and the body a greater 'plasticity' which can only be achieved by the subtle calculation of appropriate patterns of consumption akin to those expounded by health promotion.[2]

To a much greater extent than previously, today individuals with access to adequate resources can construct their own self-identities and, within limits, be the authors of their own subjectivities. Late modern self-identities are considered to be largely constituted through role-playing, image construction and the consumption of goods and services with varying identity-values (Featherstone, 1991b). Rigid modern identities determined by occupation, gender, age, race, locality and so on are thus analytically juxtaposed to emerging late modern flexible identities supposedly constructed around social practices foregrounding culture, leisure, play, technology and consumption (Kellner, 1992).

Such models can be criticised on at least two grounds. First, for taking as axiomatic access to adequate resources. For many people it is still undoubtedly the case that use-value and exchange-value retain an overwhelming priority over identity-value. As Warde (1992: 26) so clearly puts it 'people play with the signs that they can afford'. Thus, although we may well be witnessing the emergence of late modern forms of self-identity it is not a uniform transformation across the population. Some actors have a much greater autonomy to construct their identities than others. Whilst some may be able to pay for cosmetic surgery others have to wait for unacceptably long periods just for routine relief from pain and other obstacles to their daily lives. Whilst some can afford to choose extra virgin olive oil and fresh vegetables, others have to sleep in cardboard boxes on the streets and eat what food they can get. Second, although there is undoubtedly some evidence for the 'loosening' of self-identity from traditional social locations there also remains broad associations between such locations and consumption preferences, as we shall see below.

However, for late modern subjects seduced by consumer culture (Bauman, 1987) – the majority of the population – the construction of self-identity is inexorably tied up not just with consumption but also, increasingly, with the body (Featherstone, 1991a). This is so because, as Shilling (1993) explains, the body may be thought of as an *unfinished* biological and social phenomenon, which is transformed, within changing limits, as a result of its participation in society. Bodies are used as markers of distinction and in contemporary society reflexive self-identity becomes increasingly tied to the *body as a project*. The body is 'seen as an entity which is in the process of becoming; a project which should be worked at and accomplished as part of an individual's self-identity' (Shilling, 1993: 12).

This notion of a body project is based on two propositions (Shilling, 1993: 200). First, that we have the technological knowledge and ability to intervene and substantially alter the body and, second, that growing numbers of people are increasingly aware of the body as an unfinished entity which is shaped partly as a result of lifestyle choices – choices that are, for the most part, the product of consumption practices. Following Giddens (1991), Shilling argues that in a culture that is dominated by risk, uncertainty and doubt, the body has come to form a secure site over which individuals are able to exert at least some control: 'Investing in the body provides people with a means of self expression ... If one feels unable to exert control over an increasingly complex society, at least one can have some effect on the size, shape and appearance of one's body' (1993: 7). From this it follows that the corollary to late modern reflexive subjectivity is a new attitude towards the body which is witnessed, or so we shall argue, by the growth of 'health-related' consumer culture, and, although we shall not discuss it here, in the increased willingness of people to contemplate ever more radical bodily transformations through the applications of various new technologies (Deitch, 1992; Rucker *et al.*, 1993). Below, we shall examine some of these propositions in the light of patterns of consumption amongst the British middle classes – the group most often viewed as hegemonic in the promulgation of 'healthy lifestyles'.

Thus, our argument so far has been that the discourse of health promotion may most appropriately be viewed as being a central feature in the transformation of health care from one based upon dangerousness, situated in the 'clinic of the subject', to one based upon risk, dispersed in the 'epidemiological' clinic of the 'community'. This late modern 'community' increasingly refers to social spaces dominated by the cultural processes of consumption. However, consumption itself is also playing an increasingly important role in the fabrication of both self-identity and, intimately linked to this, the creation of various body projects. There is a concurrency between the political project of health promotion based upon risk calculations of the 'epidemiological' clinic and the wider cultural emergence of consumer 'healthism', the dominance of which all but engulfs the specificity of health promotion. Further, there is a clear correspondence between the techniques of the 'epidemiological' clinic in the sphere of health care and the techniques of market research in the sphere of consumer culture more generally (O'Brien, 1992; this volume). Like the distribution of health and illness, the consumption of different clusters of goods and services are clearly related to the socio-economic and demographic characteristics of the population. Knowledge of four or five key social characteristics will allow us to estimate not just individual propensities towards various characteristics associated with health, but also the likelihood of the ownership of any number of different commodities. It is this complex relationship between consumption, health and cultural context to which we now turn.

CONSUMPTION, CULTURE AND HEALTH

The sociology of consumption is usually considered to be constituted by two relatively distinct areas of work (Warde, 1990). The first, deriving from urban sociology and politics, relates to the efficacy, or otherwise, of consumption sector cleavages compared to production-based class differences, in explanations of cultural, political and social actions (see Savage and Warde (1993: 147–63) for an overview). The second, deriving from the tradition of cultural studies, is more concerned with the meaning and experience of consumption within contemporary consumer culture (Featherstone, 1991b). Whilst the first of these has already had some influence upon the sociological analysis of health and illness (Busfield, 1990; 1992; Calnan and Cant, 1992; Flynn, 1992) little has, as yet, been made of the second. In the rest of this chapter we shall attempt to indicate how work in this second tradition, especially that of Bourdieu (1984), might be utilised in order to analyse some aspect of the relationship between consumption and health in the light of our observations on the discourse of health promotion. First, we consider the consumption of drugs within the context of consumer culture, and second, summarising the work of Savage *et al.* (1992), we consider patterns of consumption amongst the British middle classes.

Bourdieu (1984) suggests that the patterning of consumption practices can best be understood in terms of what he terms the *habitus* of different social groups. This refers to the underlying pattern of unconscious preferences, classificatory schemes and taken-for-granted choices which differ between groups and distinguishes them one from the other. Bourdieu suggests that if one belongs to a certain group and identifies with that group, then one will make choices in everyday consumption rituals that reflect the habitus of this group. The habitus of any particular group thus becomes incorporated into body shape and is passed on from generation to generation by way of processes of acculturation. From this view, 'lifestyles' are seen as groupings of commodity consumption involving shared symbolic codes of stylised behaviour, adornment and taste. To understand people's consumption preferences, it is thus crucial to be aware of the symbolic meanings that are embedded within commodities and practices. The meanings associated with different commodities and lifestyle practices which the discourse of health promotion attempts to constitute thus have to compete with much stronger and deeper cultural logics (Thorogood, 1992a). This, for example, is clearly the case with the consumption and lifestyle practices associated with drug use.

Drugs of distinction: drug use in consumer culture

The most obvious cultural distinctions in drug use are the commonplace ones noted by Bourdieu in relation to the differential consumption of alcohol across gender. Data from the 1990/91 British General Household Survey (GHS) reveal significant differences in 'tastes' for different types of alcoholic drink not just in relation to gender but also across social class.[3] The data shown in Table 16.1 reveal that beer is the overwhelmingly most popular drink amongst men. Almost 50 per cent of those who drank at all said that it was the one drink that they drank the most. Next came wine and then spirits. For women wine was the drink most frequently drunk (26 per cent), followed by beer and then spirits. For men the propensity to favour beer increases as socio-economic group decreases and the propensity towards wine and spirits increases as socio-economic group increases. The pattern for beer and wine is repeated for women, but the propensity to favour spirits increases as socio-economic group decreases for women.

We might reasonably posit that such a cultural patterning will also be present in the consumption of other drugs. At the level of images if not at the level of hard data we already have some drugs of 'distinction': cocaine as the 'banker's drug'; crack, speed and solvents as the drugs of the less prosperous; ecstasy as the drug of the rave-goer; and, possibly, cannabis as the drug of students and the public sector middle classes. However, for obvious reasons we have no way of accurately measuring the patterns of consumption of illicit drugs. Legal drugs are much easier to monitor and examine, cigarettes being ideal for our purposes here.

It is clear for instance, again via a secondary analysis of 1990/91 GHS data, that in relation to gender, strong preferences for different brands of cigarette are apparent. Over 62 per cent of *Dunhill, Lambert and Butler, Silk Cut* and *Regal* cigarette smokers are women, whilst *Benson and Hedges, Embassy, Marlboro* and *Rothmans* are favoured by men. Some clear social class preferences for different brands of cigarette are also apparent. Table 16.2 shows the proportion of some selected brands of cigarettes smoked by people from different socio-economic groups. Both *Benson and Hedges* and *Silk Cut* are popular with both professionals (accounting for over 55 per cent of the category) and employers and managers (almost 40 per cent). However, their popularity decreases as socio-economic group decreases. For example, *Benson and Hedges* are

Table 16.1 Drink most frequently taken by socio-economic group of the head of household by gender for those aged 18 to 60

Males	Socio-economic group of head of household						
	1	2	3	4	5	6	7
Shandy	1.4	4.0	2.7	5.1	4.9	4.8	4.8
Beer	39.2	39.8	41.2	46.2	49.9	55.7	68.3
Spirit	6.2	7.9	5.5	5.1	5.8	3.2	2.4
Sherry	1.1	1.3	1.9	2.4	0.9	–	–
Wine	14.4	12.0	11.1	6.3	6.0	4.1	1.2
2+ types	37.8	35.0	37.6	34.7	32.5	32.3	23.4
N	439	1260	583	331	1998	663	167
Females							
Shandy	2.0	2.1	1.6	1.7	3.2	3.4	5.6
Beer	6.1	9.4	11.4	16.4	16.6	22.1	27.0
Spirit	9.9	11.7	9.2	14.0	14.6	12.8	12.8
Sherry	5.6	6.2	7.0	5.8	5.6	3.7	4.6
Wine	36.8	33.3	31.5	24.6	23.6	17.3	12.8
2+ types	39.6	37.3	39.4	37.6	36.5	40.7	37.2
N	394	1260	686	537	1876	820	196

Key

1 Professional
2 Employers and managers
3 Intermediate non-manual
4 Junior non-manual
5 Skilled manual
6 Semi-skilled manual
7 Unskilled manual

Source: GHS 1990/91 Data Files, own analysis

smoked by only 11.9 per cent of those from the unskilled manual category and *Silk Cut* by only 3.6 per cent. The popularity of other brands, such as *John Player* and *Regal*, show a social class gradient, albeit not so pronounced, in the opposite direction. For example, *John Player* is preferred by over 9 per cent of the unskilled manual category, but by only 2.4 per cent of professionals.

In addition to this clear social patterning of brands the existence of a generic aesthetic associated with cigarettes has been recognised by Klein (1993). He points to the 'sublime' quality of consuming such a fateful commodity knowing that it will damage one's health if not kill. This aspect is central to the contemporary mystique of the cigarette and no doubt the reason why *Death Cigarettes* have sold so well. This brand of cigarette highlights the imminent danger of smoking, along with a black packet and a skull and crossbones as their emblem. This clever marketing

Table 16.2 Percentage of smokers who smoke selected brands of cigarette by socio-economic group (SEG)

SEG	Brand of cigarette				Total
	Benson and Hedges	*Silk Cut*	*John Player*	*Regal*	
Professional	21.7	33.7	2.4	1.2	83
Employers and managers	19.9	19.1	7.5	1.4	492
Intermediate non-manual	17.3	19.8	9.3	3.1	450
Junior non-manual	19.8	16.6	6.6	3.8	737
Skilled manual	18.7	8.1	7.6	3.4	1031
Semi-skilled manual	15.5	8.6	8.8	5.2	946
Unskilled manual	11.9	3.6	9.4	4.7	278

Source: GHS 1990/91 Data Files, own analysis

strategy makes sense only because they are consumed as cultural objects – they are not qualitatively superior to other brands. Cigarette advertising provides a rich source for analyses of the 'grammar' of distinction. Branding deliberately creates and exploits differences using market segmentation techniques and targeting specific types of smokers – 'Marlboro Men', 'Kim Women', etc. We can see in such advertisements the translation from routine everyday gesture to the creation of brand images. Cigarettes are intimately implicated in the aesthetics of everyday life and fashion (Amos, 1992). This is indicated by the recent attention of 'style leaders' to cigarettes. Smoking was introduced to the cat-walk by models in Paris in 1993 as part of Gianfranco Ferres' collection for Dior, showing the cigarette to advantage as a fashion accessory. Style magazines also occasionally run articles – sometimes far richer in sociological insight than much health promotion research – in appreciation of the stylish versatility of smoking and its expressive quality (Bracewell and Wilde, 1990) as shown in Figure 16.2.[4]

The consumption of cigarettes is thus clearly not just related to their addictive qualities. They also play an important cultural function in the habitus of a range of different social groups. They are used in important ritualistic and expressive ways that have little to do with any consideration of the health risks associated with their consumption.

However, having said this, the 'risky' qualities of smoking (and other drug use) also have their attractions. Data from the 1990/91 GHS suggests that the great majority of people are aware of the health risks associated with smoking. Nevertheless many people continue to smoke and use other drugs in full knowledge of the risks. This is because, as we have already indicated, risks themselves hold a certain attraction. Risk taking amongst young people is often portrayed as a commonplace behavioural characteristic and one that spans a number of activities including drug use, unsafe sexual behaviour and other dangerous activities (Plant and Plant, 1992). Reasons have been put forward for the greater extent of risk taking amongst the poor and disadvantaged – those with poor or no housing, high levels of unemployment, low incomes, fragmented family structures

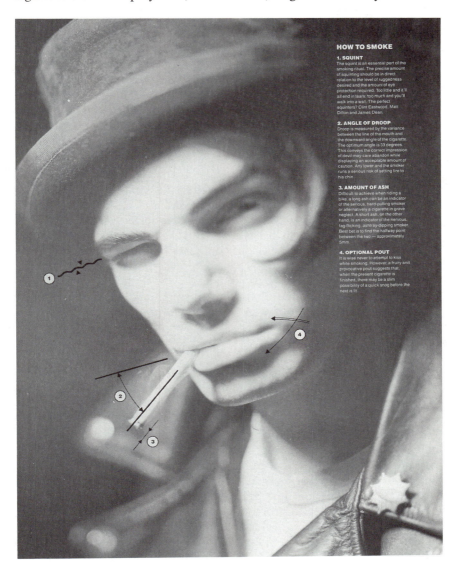

Figure 16.2 How to smoke
Source: Blitz Magazine, 86, February 1990

and stressful life events. What is not considered in these accounts however is that there might be a high cultural value in risk behaviour, or at least in risk presentation through consumption. The currency of risk can be gained by the consumption of certain drugs. Drug capital (both cultural and physical) can, in Bourdieu's terms, then be exchanged for other sorts of capital. There is then a certain cachet in assuming certain drug lifestyles. The adoption of cocaine by yuppies in the 1980s may be consistent with their image as 'heroic consumers' open to the adventure and exoticness of other cultures and sub-cultures (see below). Equally, the drug shaped body might be a form of physical capital that can only be achieved through drug use – the emaciated, stereotyped face of the heroin or amphetamine user, the 'beer gut' of the beer drinker, the wrinkled eyes of the smoker or the inflated muscles of the steroid-using body builder, are all examples of drug-associated physical capital.

Clearly there are much more obvious economic reasons for the use and sale of drugs by deprived groups. On the other hand, those with least economic capital may be most in need of other forms of capital. The value of drug consumption might therefore be stratified by income in ways that are not determined by purely economic considerations. Drugs then can be analysed as *risk products* that act as social distinguishers. The cultural market for certain drugs and the calculus of risk involved thus provides an example of a powerful countervailing force to the discourse of health promotion operating at consumption sites. Indeed, it is clearly possible that some prevention campaigns may have the unintended function of increasing the value of certain drugs by invoking a recalibration in the rates of exchange between risks and cultural capital.

Middle class consumption patterns

The relationship between lifestyle, habitus and patterns of consumption has also recently been explored amongst the British middle classes by Savage *et al.* (1992: 99–158). Their work is based upon a secondary analysis of data collected by the British Market Research Bureau (BMRB) for 1987 and 1988 on some 11,000 'middle class' adults. Their analysis suggests some clear associations between patterns of consumption associated with health and a range of different variables. These associations are important not just because of the hegemonic role the middle classes play in opinion formation, but also because it is from the middle classes that health promotion professionals derive. This emergent group function as 'cultural intermediaries' (Featherstone, 1991b) in the dissemination of the norms, values and practices associated with 'healthy living'.

High incomes are strongly associated with consumption practices associated with health and body maintenance. However, high incomes are also

– and perversely – strongly associated with consumption marked by excess and indulgence, especially eating and drinking. It is also clear that those on low(er) incomes are largely excluded from both forms of consumption. Thus, for some groups in the middle class consumption is not organised into the form of a lifestyle marked by any single coherent organising principle – high extravagance goes hand in hand with a culture of health and body maintenance. Savage *et al.* – with tongue in cheek – term this a *postmodern* lifestyle.

People with high cultural capital but low economic capital who are largely reliant on the state for employment – those in education, health and welfare – demonstrate patterns of consumption marked by clear *ascetic* principles. This group has a high propensity towards climbing, skating, table tennis, hiking and yoga and appears to be drawn towards a culture of 'authenticity' and the 'natural' (Urry, 1990). This group also displays a below average consumption of alcohol and below average participation in 'sports' such as snooker and fishing. They have a below average membership of health clubs – probably a function of the cost of such membership and their preference for the authentic over simulations/ simulcra – and a low propensity towards participation in team games and organised collective sports. They have a high propensity towards a range of outdoor activities – camping, multi-centre country and mountain holidays and so on – and display some interest in 'high culture': they are more likely to go to plays, classical concerts and contemporary dance events than the middle class as a whole. Savage *et al.* suggest that this ascetic lifestyle is associated with a habitus reflecting both the group's 'expert knowledge' of the self and the body and its relative insulation from the world of private business. It is – at one and the same time – a habitus marked by both the rejection of competitive individualism *and* a rationalisation of the reality of relatively low incomes.

Workers in local and central government – civil servants rather than welfare workers – differ again in terms of their consumption patterns from other members of the middle classes. They have very little in the way of 'distinctive' patterns of consumption – with the exception of a taste for bowls and a hatred of squash in their sporting activities. They tend to lead very *conventional* lifestyles. They tend to inhabit relatively closed worlds, and have a high commitment to their careers (as they are largely reliant upon organisational assets rather than cultural or economic capital) compared to their families.[5]

The data also demonstrate some interesting differences in the lifestyles and consumption practices of those who left school at 16 compared to those who completed their education at 21–3 or 24 and over. If we assume that these different educational leaving points represent an ordinal scale of cultural capital, as manifest in educational qualifications (no degree, first degree, postgraduate), then a clear association is revealed between levels of such capital and the propensity to engage in various forms of 'body culture' associated with keeping fit and healthy. Those with degrees also tend to combine such 'body culture' with 'non-English' tastes – having a particular liking for non-English food (especially French, Chinese, Middle Eastern and Indian), holidays in Western Europe in 'sophisticated' localities and mineral water. Those with postgraduate experience are distinct again from those with just first degrees in their taste for 'high culture', especially opera, classical concerts and art galleries. They also have a higher propensity for climbing. They are not at all keen on competitive sports and more hedonistic – 'Californian' – modes of consumption. Those with postgraduate qualifications share then, to some extent, the tastes of the less well-educated upper classes – including the aristocracy.

The propensity for health-related consumption is, as we have seen, widening its social base from the middle classes as it becomes more and more emblematic of late modern subjectivity and its associated body projects. As advanced economies become increasingly concerned with the circulation of capital through information, symbols and signs, the process of reflexive modernisation (Lash and Urry, 1994) demands that cultural assets become more important for everyone, not just for those with a social base in education, health, welfare and cultural occupations. However, it is this group that has been at the 'vanguard' of changes in lifestyle and consumption patterns more generally. The asceticism of the group, which was, in part, a function of their low economic assets, is gradually becoming incorporated within lifestyles more fully participating in the materialism of consumer culture. However, this adoption of a healthy lifestyle by the more materialistically minded has not been via a process of 'replacement' – rather it now 'sits beside' other forms of consumption to be 'sampled' as part of the postmodern pastiche identified in the pattern of the consumption of those with high incomes. The reasons for this we have already discussed; the late modern world is 'a runaway world' where 'not only is the pace of social change much faster than in any prior system' so is its 'scope and . . . profoundness' (Giddens, 1991: 16). Thus, ontological insecurity pushes people towards engagements with aspects of their lives they perceive they might be able to display some control over, prime amongst which is the body.

In this section we have examined the manner in which the discourse of health promotion has been incorporated within the lifestyles and consumption preferences of the middle classes. For one fraction of the class – the *ascetics*, some of whom may well work in the health promotion industry – the discourse represents simply a widening of their own world views and practices. Although there is some evidence that aspects of the *ascetics'* 'healthy lifestyle' is widening its appeal to other members of the class it is clear that it is being substantially mediated by the specificities of their preexisting cultural preferences.

CONCLUDING COMMENTS

In this chapter we have explored various aspects of the relationship between health promotion and 'health-related' consumer culture. To understand the emergence of current health promotion it is necessary to situate it within contemporary consumption practices. Important aspects of its work only make sense in relation to late modern consumer culture. Our argument has been that the 'epidemiological' clinic of late modern medicine seeks to regulate collective health status via invoking changes in individual patterns of consumption. It does this by reliance on a wide range of market-oriented behavioural research, though it has largely neglected cultural analyses of the processes of change it seeks to bring about. If it is to succeed in influencing consumption in the ways it desires it will have to consider such cultural aspects more seriously than it has done hitherto. At the moment the new public health relies too heavily upon models of health promotion efficacy derived from individualistic models of health behaviour. Although these models have been rightly criticised for ignoring social structural constraints upon such behaviours (Nettleton and Bunton, this volume), our argument here has been that culture also plays a crucial role in the determination of people's tastes and preferences. Drawing upon Bourdieu's work we have attempted to illustrate how such analysis might proceed. There are clearly a great many more directions such a study might and should take. To the extent that we are going to rely more and more upon health promotion as the main means of governing health and illness we need to come to terms more directly with this cultural dimension of consumption and health.

NOTES

1 On the notion of late modernism see Giddens (1990; 1991), Hall *et al.* (1992) and Wagner (1994). Despite our use of such a simplistic and polarised ideal type we still prefer this term to the ubiquitous 'postmodernism' (Kelly and Charlton, this volume), which is suggestive of a more fundamental binary shift in social and cultural processes than is allowed for by current evidence. All too often distinctions that are analytically useful become reified as empirical categories.

2 The recent analysis of the 'consuming body' offered by Falk (1994) offers a number of sociological insights into this and related issues.

3 Material from the GHS was made available through the OPCS and the ESRC Data Archive with the permission of the Controller of H.M. Stationery Office. For further details see Burrows and Nettleton (1995).

4 Thanks are due to Amanda Amos for alerting us to this material.

5 It would be interesting to discover if these patterns of consumption are altering

with the advent of the new managerialism in the public sector which increasingly draws upon both the rhetoric and organisational form of private sector companies. For example, Quarry House in Leeds, the location of the NHS Executive and the Benefits Agency, includes facilities such as a swimming pool, squash courts and a gym for its staff.

References

Action on Smoking and Health (ASH) (1989) *Passive Smoking*, Factsheet 7, London: ASH.

Action on Smoking and Health (ASH) (1993) *It Affects us All*, Information Sheet, London: ASH.

Action on Smoking and Health (ASH) Women and Smoking Group (1993) *Her Share of Misfortune: Women, Smoking and Low Income*, London: ASH.

Ahmad, W. I. U. (ed.) (1993a) *'Race' and Health in Contemporary Britain*, Buckingham: Open University Press.

Ahmad, W. I. U (1993b) 'Promoting Equitable Health and Health Care: A Case for Action' in W. I. U Ahmad (ed.) *'Race' and Health in Contemporary Britain*, Buckingham: Open University Press.

Aird, V. (1986) *Whiteway Health Project Annual Report*, Bath: Whiteway Health Project.

Amos, A. (1992) *Style and Image: Tobacco and Alcohol Images*, London: Health Education Authority.

Amos, V. and Parmar, P. (1984) 'Challenging Imperial Feminism', *Feminist Review*, 17, 2–19, July.

Anderson, D. (ed.) (1986) *A Diet of Reason*, London: Social Affairs Unit.

Anderson, J., Huppert, F. and Rose, G. (1993) 'Normality, Deviance and Minor Psychiatric Morbidity in the Community: A Population-Based Approach to General Health Questionnaire Data in the Health and Lifestyle Survey', *Psychological Medicine*, 23, 2, 475–85.

Anderson, R. (1983) *Health Promotion: An Overview*, Technical Paper Prepared for WHO, Copenhagen: WHO Regional Office for Europe.

Andres, R. (1980) 'Effect of Obesity on Total Mortality', *International Journal of Obesity*, 4, 381–6.

Anthias, F. and Yuval-Davis, N. (1983) 'Contextualising Feminism – Gender, Ethnic and Class Divisions', *Feminist Review*, 15, 62–75, November.

Antonovsky, A. (1985) *Health, Stress and Coping*, San Francisco: Josey Bass.

Antonovsky, A. (1987) *Unravelling the Mystery of Health*, San Francisco: Josey Bass.

Armstrong, D. (1983) *Political Anatomy of the Body: Medical Knowledge in Britain in the Twentieth Century*, Cambridge: Cambridge University Press.

Armstrong, D. (1993a) 'From Clinical Gaze to a Regime of Total Health' in A. Beattie, M. Gott, L. Jones and L. Sidell (eds) *Health and Wellbeing: A Reader*, London: Macmillan.

Armstrong, D. (1993b) 'Public Health Spaces and the Fabrication of Identity', *Sociology*, 27, 3, 393–410.

Min o) H?

Armstrong, P. (1982) 'The Myth of Meeting Needs in Adult Education and Community Development', *Critical Social Policy*, 2, 2, 24–37.

Arney, W. R. and Bergen, B. (1984) *Medicine and the Management of Living: Taming the Last Great Beast*, London: Chicago Press.

Aronow, W. S. (1978) 'Effect of Passive Smoking on Angina Pectoris', *New England Journal of Medicine*, 299, 1, 21–24.

ARP (Association of Retired Persons) 050, Reporter (1993), 19, Summer.

Ashton, J. (1988) 'Health Promotion and the Concept of Community' in R. Anderson, J. Davies, I. Kickbusch, D. McQueen and R. Turner (eds) *Health Behaviour Research and Health Promotion*, Oxford: Oxford University Press.

Ashton, J. and Seymour, H. (1988) *The New Public Health*, Milton Keynes: Open University Press.

Australian Health Ministers' Advisory Council (1988) *Health for All Australians*, Sydney: Commonwealth Department of Community Services and Health.

Backett, K. (1992) 'The Construction of Health Knowledge in Middle Class Families', *Health Education Research: Theory and Practice*, 7, 4, 497–507.

Backett, K., Davison, C. and Mullen, K. (1994) 'Lay Evaluation of Health and Healthy Lifestyles: Evidence from Three Studies', *British Journal of General Practice*, 44, 277–80.

Baggot, R. (1991) 'Looking Forward to the Past? The Politics of Public Health', *Journal of Social Policy*, 20, 2, 191–213.

Bakalar, J. and Grinspoon, L. (1984) *Drug Control in a Free Society*, Cambridge: Cambridge University Press.

Balarajan, R. and Raleigh, S. (1993) *Ethnicity and Health: A Guide for the NHS*, London: Department of Health.

Baldwin, S. and Twigg, J. (1991) 'Women and Community Care: Reflections on a Debate' in M. Maclean and D. Groves (eds) *Women's Issues in Social Policy*, London: Routledge.

Balint, M. (1957) *The Doctor, His Patient and the Illness*, Tunbridge Wells: Pitman Medical.

Balshem, M. (1991) 'Cancer, Control and Causality – Talking About Cancer in a Working-Class Community', *American Ethnologist*, 18, 1, 152–72.

Barker, D. J. P. (ed.) (1992) *Fetal and Infant Origins of Adult Disease*, London: British Medical Journal.

Barnes, B. and Shapin, S. (eds) (1979) *Natural Order*, London: Sage.

Bartley, M. (1985) 'Coronary Heart Disease and the Public Health 1850–1983', *Sociology of Health and Illness*, 7, 3, 289–313.

Bartley, M. (1990) 'Do We Need a Strong Programme in Medical Sociology?', *Sociology of Health and Illness*, 12, 4, 371–90.

Baudrillard, J. (1981) *For a Critique of the Political Economy of the Sign*, St Louis: Telos Press.

Bauman, Z. (1987) *Legislators and Interpreters: On Modernity, Postmodernity and Intellectuals*, Cambridge: Polity Press.

Bauman, Z. (1992a) *Intimations of Post-Modernity*, London: Routledge.

Bauman, Z. (1992b) *Mortality, Immortality and Other Life Strategies*, Cambridge: Polity.

Beattie, A. (1991) 'Knowledge and Control in Health Promotion: A Test Case for Social Policy and Social Theory' in J. Gabe, M. Calnan and M. Bury (eds) *The Sociology of the Health Service*, London: Routledge.

Beck, U. (1992a) *Risk Society: Towards a New Modernity*, London: Sage.

Beck, U. (1992b) 'From Industrial Society to Risk Society: Questions of Survival,

Social Structure and Ecological Enlightenment' in M. Featherstone (ed.) *Cultural Theory and Cultural Change*, London: Sage.

Beer, S. (1982) *Britain Against Itself*, London: Faber and Faber.

Belfer, M., Mulliken, B. and Cochran, T. (1979) 'Cosmetic Surgery as an Antecedent to Life Change', *American Journal of Psychiatry*, 136, 199–201.

bell hooks (1991) *Yearning: Race, Gender and Cultural Politics*, London: Turnaround.

Bennett, P and Hodgson, R. (1992) 'Psychology and Health Promotion' in R. Bunton and G. MacDonald (eds) *Health Promotion: Disciplines and Diversity*, London: Routledge.

Berscheid, E. and Gangestad, S. (1982) 'The Social Psychological Implications of Facial Physical Attractiveness', *Clinics in Plastic Surgery*, 9, 289–95.

Bertaux, D. (1983) 'Vie Quotidienne ou Modes de Vie?' ['Everyday Life or Lifestyles?'], *Revue Suisse de Sociologie*, 9, 1, 67–83.

Biggs, S. (1993) *Understanding Ageing: Images, Attitudes and Professional Practice*, Buckingham: Open University Press.

Blackburn, C. and Graham, H. (1993) *Smoking Among Working Class Mothers: Information Pack*, Warwick: University of Warwick.

Blackburn, H. *et al.* (1984) 'The Minnessota Heart Health Programme: A Research and Development Project in Cardiovascular Disease Prevention' in J. Mattazaro *et al.* (eds) *Rural Health: A Handbook of Health Enhancement Disease Prevention*, New York: John Wiley and Sons.

Blaxter, M. (1990) *Health and Lifestyles*, London: Routledge.

Boissevain, J. (1974) 'Towards a Sociology of Social Anthropology', *Theory and Society*, 1, 211–30.

Bourdieu, P. (1984) *Distinction: A Social Critique of the Judgement of Taste*, London: Routledge.

Bracewell, M. and Wilde, J. (1990) 'Smoking is Good for You', *Blitz Magazine*, 86, 606–15, February.

Breeze, E., Trevor. G. and Wilmot, A. (1991) *General Household Survey, 1989*, London: Office of Population and Census Surveys.

Broadcasting Support Services (1991) *Smokers Can Harm Your Health*, Transcript of BBC *Horizon* Programme, 21 January, London: BBC.

Brody, J. (1987) 'Research Lifts Blame from Many of the Obese', *The New York Times*, 24 March.

Broverman, I. K. *et al.* (1970) 'Sex Role Stereotypes and Clinical Judgements of Mental Health', *Journal of Consultant Psychology*, 34, 1, 1–7.

Brown, C. (1984) *Black and White Britain: The Third PSI Survey*, London: Heinemann.

Brown, P. (1992) 'Popular Epidemiology and Toxic Waste Contamination: Lay and Professional Ways of Knowing', *Journal of Health and Social Behaviour*, 33, 267–81.

Brown, P. and Scase, R. (eds) (1991) *Poor Work: Disadvantage and the Division of Labour*, Milton Keynes: Open University Press.

Bryan, B., Dadzie, S. and Scafe, S. (1985) *The Heart of the Race: Black Women's Lives in Britain*, London, Virago.

Bryant, J. H. (1988) 'Health for All: The Dream and the Reality', *World Health Forum*, 9.

Bunton, R. (1990) 'Regulating Our Favourite Drug' in P. Abbott and G. Payne (eds) *New Directions in the Sociology of Health*, London: Falmer.

Bunton, R. (1991) 'Marketing the Social: Postmodern Tendencies in Health

Promotion', Paper Presented to the British Sociological Association Annual Conference on 'Health and Society', Manchester, April.

Bunton, R. (1992a) 'Health Promotion as Social Policy' in R. Bunton and G. MacDonald (eds) *Health Promotion: Disciplines and Diversity*, London: Routledge.

Bunton, R. (1992b) 'More Than a Woolly Jumper: Health Promotion as Social Regulation', *Critical Public Health*, 3, 2, 4–11.

Bunton, R. and MacDonald, G. (eds) (1992) *Health Promotion: Disciplines and Diversity*, London: Routledge.

Bunton, R., Murphey, S. and Bennett, P. (1991) 'Theories of Behavioural Change and their Use in Health Promotion', *Health Education Research: Theory and Practice*, 6, 2, 153–62.

Burrows, R. and Nettleton, S. (1995) 'Going Against the Grain: An Analysis of Smoking and "Heavy" Drinking Amongst the British Middle Classes', *Sociology of Health and Illness* (in press).

Bury, J. (1994) 'Women and HIV/AIDS: Medical Issues' in L. Doyal, J. Naidoo and T. Wilton (eds) *Women and AIDS: Setting a Feminist Agenda*, London: Taylor and Francis.

Busfield, J. (1990) 'Sectoral Divisions in Consumption: The Case of Medical Care', *Sociology*, 24, 1, 77–96.

Busfield, J. (1992) 'Medicine and Markets: Power, Choice and the Consumption of Private Medical Care' in R. Burrows and C. Marsh (eds) *Consumption and Class: Divisions and Change*, London: Macmillan.

Butler, R. N. (1969) 'Age-Ism: Another Form of Bigotry', *The Gerontologist*, 9, 243–6.

Byrd, J. C., Shapiro, R. S. and Scheidermayer, D. L. (1989) 'Passive Smoking: A Review of the Medical and Legal Issues', *American Journal of Public Health*, 79, 2, 209–15.

Cahnman, W. (1968) 'The Stigma of Obesity', *The Sociological Quarterly*, 9, 283–99.

Calnan, M. (1984) 'The Health Belief Model and Participation in Programmes for the Early Detection of Breast Cancer: A Comparative Analysis', *Social Science and Medicine*, 19, 823–30.

Calnan, M. (1987) *Health and Illness: The Lay Perspective*, London: Tavistock.

Calnan, M. (1991) *Preventing Coronary Heart Disease: Prospects, Policies and Politics*, London: Routledge.

Calnan, M. and Cant, S. (1992) 'Principles and Practice: The Case of Private Health Insurance' in R. Burrows and C. Marsh (eds) *Consumption and Class: Divisions and Change*, London: Macmillan.

Calnan, M., Cant, S. and Gabe, J. (1993) *Going Private: Why People Pay for their Health Care*, Buckingham: Open University Press.

CAPT (Child Accident Prevention Trust) (1989) *Basic Principles of Child Accident Prevention: A Guide to Action*, London: CAPT.

Carter, Y. H. and Jones, P. W. (1993) 'Accidents Among Children Under Five Years Old: A General Practice Based Study in North Staffordshire', *British Journal of General Practice*, 43, 159–63.

Cash, T., Winstead, B. and Janda, H. (1986) 'The Great American Shape-Up', *Psychology Today*, 20, 30–34 April.

Castel, R. (1991) 'From Dangerousness to Risk' in G. Burchell, C. Gordon and P. Miller (eds) *The Foucault Effect: Studies in Governmentality*, London: Harvester Wheatsheaf.

Castells, M. (1977) *The Urban Question*, London: Edward Arnold.

Catford, J. C. (1983) 'Positive Health Indicators – Towards New Information Bases for Health Promotion', *Community Medicine*, 5, 125–32.

Catford, J. C. and Parish, R. (1989) ' "Heartbeat Wales": New Horizons for Health Promotion in the Community – The Philosophy of Heartbeat Wales' in D. Seedhouse and A. Cribb (eds) *Changing Ideas in Health Care*, London: John Wiley and Sons.

Chapman, S., Borland, R., Hill, D., Owen, N. and Woodward S. (1990) 'Why the Tobacco Industry Fears the Passive Smoking Issue', *International Journal of Health Services*, 20, 3, 417–27.

Chapman, S. and Egger, G. (1983) 'Myth in Cigarette Advertising and Health Promotion' in H. Davis and P. Walton (eds) *Language, Image and Media*, Oxford: Blackwell.

Charles, N. (1993) *Gender Divisions and Social Change*, Brighton: Harvester Wheatsheaf.

Charles, N. and Kerr, M. (1986) 'Issues of Responsibility and Control in the Feeding of Families' in S. Rodmell and A. Watt (eds) *The Politics of Health Education*, London: Routledge and Kegan Paul.

Charles, N. and Kerr, M. (1987) 'Just the Way it Is: Gender and Age Differences in Family Food Consumption' in M. Brannen and G. Wilson (eds) *Give and Take in Families*, London: Allen and Unwin.

Charles, N. and Kerr, M. (1988) *Women, Food and Families*, Manchester: Manchester University Press.

Charlton, B. G. (1993a) 'The Health Obsession', *The Salisbury Review*, March, 31–5, March.

Charlton, B. G. (1993b) 'Public Health Medicine – a Different Kind of Ethics', *Journal of the Royal Society of Medicine*, 86, 497–9.

Charlton, B. G. (1994) 'Is Inequality Bad for the National Health?', *Lancet*, 343, 221–2.

Cliff, K. S. (1984) *Accidents: Causes, Prevention and Services*, London: Croom Helm.

Cohen, R. and Schnelle, T. (eds) (1986) *Cognition and Fact – Materials on Ludwig Fleck*, Dordrecht: D. Reidel Publishing.

Cohen, S. (1973) *Folk Devils and Moral Panics*, London: Paladin.

Cohen, S. (1985) *Visions of Social Control: Crime, Punishment and Classification*, Cambridge: Polity Press.

Cole, T. R. (1992) *The Journey of Life: A Cultural History of Ageing in America*, Cambridge: Cambridge University Press.

Cole-Hamilton, I. (1987) 'Food and Poverty in the 1980s', *Radical Community Medicine*, 29, 37–9.

Colley, J. R. T., Holland, W. W. and Corkhill, R. T. (1974) 'Influences of Passive Smoking and Parental Phlegm on Pneumonia and Bronchitis in Early Childhood', *Lancet*, November 2, ii, 1031–4.

Conrad, P. and Walsh, D. (1992) 'The New Corporate Work Ethic: Lifestyle and the Control of Work', *International Journal of Health Services*, 22, 1, 89–111.

Coreil, J. and Levin, J. S. (1984) 'A Critique of the Lifestyle Concept in Public Health Education', *International Quarterly of Community Health and Education*, 5, 2, 103–14.

Cornwell, J. (1984) *Hard-Earned Lives: Accounts of Health and Illness from East London*, London: Tavistock.

Crawford, R. (1977) 'You are Dangerous to Your Health: The Politics and Ideology of Victim Blaming', *International Journal of Health Services*, 7, 4, 663–80.

Crawford, R. (1980) 'Healthism and the Medicalization of Everyday Life', *International Journal of Health Services*, 10, 3, 365–88.

Crawford, R. (1984) 'A Cultural Account of "Health": Control, Release, and the Social Body' in J. McKinlay (ed) *Issues in the Political Economy of Health Care*, London: Tavistock.

Crawford, R. (1986) 'Individual Responsibility and Health Politics' in P. Conrad and R. Kern (eds) *The Sociology of Health and Illness: Critical Perspectives*, New York: St Martin's Press.

Croft, A. and Sibert, J. (1992) 'Accident Prevention – Environmental Change and Education' in J. Sibert (ed.) *Accidents and Emergencies in Childhood*, London: Royal College of Physicians.

Crook, S., Pakulski, R. and Waters, M. (1992) *Postmodernization: Changes in Advanced Society*, London: Sage.

Daly, M. (1979) *Gyn/Ecology: The Meta Ethics of Radical Feminism*, London: Women's Press.

Dankmeijer, P. (1993) 'The Construction of Identities as a Means of Survival: The Case of Gay and Lesbian Teachers', *Journal of Homosexuality*, 24, 3/4, 95–105.

Davey Smith, G. (1993) 'Review of *Smoking – Making the Risky Decision* by W. K. Viscusi', *Lancet*, 341, 1523–4.

Davey Smith, G., Bartley, M. and Blane, D. (1990) 'The Black Report on Socio-economic Inequalities in Health 10 Years On', *British Medical Journal*, 301, 373–7.

Davey Smith, G. and Shipley, M. J. (1991) 'Confounding of Occupation and Smoking: Its Magnitude and Consequences', *Social Science and Medicine*, 32, 1297–1300.

Davies, J. and Kelly, M. (eds) (1993) *Healthy Cities: Research and Practice*, London: Routledge.

Davis, B. and French, W. A. (1989) 'Exploring Advertising Usage Segments Among the Aged', *Journal of Advertising Research*, 29, 1, 22–9.

Davison, C., Davey Smith, G. and Frankel, S. (1991) 'Lay Epidemiology and the Prevention Paradox: The Implications of Coronary Candidacy for Health Education', *Sociology of Health and Illness*, 13, 1, 1–19.

Davison, C., Frankel, S. and Davey Smith, G. (1992) 'The Limits of Lifestyle: Re-assessing "Fatalism" in the Popular Culture of Illness Prevention', *Social Science and Medicine*, 34, 6, 675–85.

Dawkins, R. (1988) *The Blind Watchmaker*, London: Penguin.

Deitch, J. (1992) *Post-Human*, Amsterdam: Idea Books.

Department of Health (1991) *The Health of the Nation*, Consultative Document, London: HMSO.

Department of Health (1992a) *The Health of the Nation: A Strategy for Health in England*, London: HMSO.

Department of Health (1992b) *The Health of the Nation . . . And You*, London: HMSO.

Department of Health (1993a) *Working Together for Better Health*, London: HMSO.

Department of Health (1993b) *AIDS – HIV Infected Health Care Workers: Guidance on the Management of Infected Health Care Workers*, Department of Health, April.

Department of Health and Social Security (DHSS) (1976a) *Prevention and Health: Everybody's Business*, London: HMSO.

Department of Health and Social Security (DHSS) (1976b) *Priorities for Health and Personal Social Services in England*, London: HMSO.

Department of Health and Social Security (DHSS) (1981) *Care in Action: A Handbook of Policies and Priorities for the Health and Personal Social Services in England*, London: HMSO.

Department of Health and Social Security (DHSS) (1986) *Primary Health Care: An Agenda for Discussion*, London: HMSO.

Department of Health and Social Security (DHSS) (1992) *Registrar General Northern Ireland, Seventieth Annual Report 1991*, Belfast: HMSO.

Department of Health and the Welsh Office (1989) *General Practice in the National Health Service – A New Contract*, London: HMSO.

Department of Transport (1985) *Compulsory Seat Belt Wearing*, London: HMSO.

Doll, R. and Hill A. B. (1950) 'Smoking and Carcinoma of the Lung', *British Medical Journal*, 30, 739–48.

Donohew, L., Palmgreen, P. and Rayburn, J. D. (1987) 'Social and Psychological Origins of Media Use: A Lifestyle Analysis', *Journal of Broadcasting and Electronic Media*, 31, 3, 255–78.

Donovan, J. (1984) 'Ethnicity and Health', *Social Science and Medicine*, 19, 7, 663–70.

Douglas, J. (1987) *Caribbean Food and Diet*, Cambridge: National Extension College.

Douglas, J. (1992) 'Black Women's Health Matters: Putting Black Women on the Research Agenda' in H. Roberts (ed.) *Women's Health Matters*, London: Routledge.

Douglas, M. (1984) *Purity and Danger: An Analysis of the Concepts of Pollution and Taboo*, London: Ark.

Douglas, M. and Isherwood, B. (1979) *A World of Goods*, New York: Basic Books.

Doyal, L. (1991) 'Promoting Women's Health' in B. Badura and I. Kickbusch (eds) *Health Promotion Research*, Copenhagen: WHO.

Doyal, L. (1994) 'Changing Medicine: Gender and the Politics of Health Care' in J. Gabe, D. Kelleher and G. Williams (eds) *Challenging Medicine*, London: Routledge.

Doyal, L. (1995) *What Makes Women Sick? Gender and the Political Economy of Health*, Basingstoke: Macmillan.

Doyal, L. with Pennell, I. (1979) *The Political Economy of Health*, London: Pluto Press.

Draper, P. (1991) *Health Through Public Policy: The Greening of Public Health*, London: Greenprint.

Dull, D. and West, C. (1987) 'The Price of Perfection: A Study of the Relations Between Women and Plastic Surgeons', Paper Presented at the Meetings of the American Sociological Association.

Durkheim, E. (1915) *The Elementary Forms of the Religious Life* (Translated by J. Ward Swaine), London: George Allen and Unwin.

Durkheim, E. (1933) *The Division of Labour in Society* (Translated by G. Simpson), New York: Free Press.

Durkheim, E. (1952) *Suicide: A Study in Sociology* (Translated by J. Spaulding and G. Simpson), London: Routledge.

Ehrenreich, J. (1978) *The Cultural Crisis of Modern Medicine*, New York: Monthly Review Press.

Ehrenreich, B. and English, D. (1973) *Complaints and Disorders: The Sexual Politics of Sickness*, New York: Writers and Readers.

Elias, N. (1971) 'The Sociology of Knowledge: New Perspectives – 1 and 2', *Sociology*, 5, 149–68 and 355–70.

Elias, N. (1978) *What Is Sociology?*, London: Hutchinson.

Elias, N. (1985) *The Loneliness of The Dying*, Oxford: Basil Blackwell.

Eriksen, M. P., LeMaistre, C. A. and Newell, G. R. (1988) 'The Health Hazards of Passive Smoking', *Annual Review of Public Health*, 9, 47–70.

Esteban, E. (1993) 'World First for HIV-Proof Spacesuits', *Gay Scotland*, 68, 22, May.

Ewles, L. (1993) 'Hope Against Hype', *Health Service Journal* 26 August, 30–1.

Exter, T. (1987) 'Lifestyle Economics: Consumer Behaviour in a Turbulent World', *American Demographics*, 9.

Falk, P. (1994) *The Consuming Body*, London: Sage.

Fannin, R. (1986) 'Shape Up!', *Marketing and Media Decisions*, February, 54–60.

Farrant, W. (1991) 'Addressing the Contradictions: Health Promotion and Community Health Action in the United Kingdom', *International Journal of Health Services*, 21, 3, 423–39.

Farrant, W. and Russell, J. (1986) *The Politics of Health Information*, London: Health Education Council.

Featherstone, M. (1987) 'Lifestyle and Consumer Culture', *Theory, Culture and Society*, 4, 1, 55–70.

Featherstone, M. (1988) 'In Pursuit of the Post-Modern: An Introduction', *Theory, Culture and Society*, 5, 2/3, 195–215.

Featherstone, M. (1991a) 'The Body in Consumer Culture' in M. Featherstone, M. Hepworth and B. S. Turner (eds) *The Body: Social Process and Cultural Theory*, London: Sage.

Featherstone, M. (1991b) *Consumer Culture and Postmodernism*, London: Sage.

Featherstone, M. and Hepworth, M. (1986) 'New Lifestyles for Old Age' in C. Phillipson (ed.) *Dependency and Independency in Old Age*, London: Croom Helm.

Featherstone, M. and Hepworth, M. (1990) 'Images of Aging' in J. Bond and P. Coleman (eds) *An Introduction to Social Gerontology*, London: Sage.

Featherstone, M. and Hepworth, M. (1991) 'The Mask of Aging' in M. Featherstone, M. Hepworth and B. S. Turner (eds) *The Body: Social Process and Cultural Theory*, London: Sage.

Featherstone, M., and Hepworth, M. (1993) 'Images of Ageing' in J. Bond, P. Coleman and S. Peace (eds) *Ageing in Society: An Introduction to Social Gerontology*, London: Sage.

Featherstone, M., Hepworth, M. and Turner, B. S. (eds) (1991) *The Body: Social Process and Cultural Theory*, London: Sage.

Finch, J. (1984) 'Community Care: Developing Non Sexist Alternatives', *Critical Social Policy*, 9, 6–18.

Fisher, S. (1986) *Development and Structure of the Body Image*, New Jersey: Erlbaum.

Fleck, L. (1979) *Genesis and Development of a Scientific Fact*, Chicago and London: University of Chicago Press.

Fleck, L. (1986a) 'On the Crisis of Reality' in R. S. Cohen and T. Schnelle (eds) *Cognition and Fact – Materials on Ludwig Fleck*, Dordrecht: D. Reidel Publishing.

Fleck, L. (1986b) 'To Look, To See, To Know' in R. S. Cohen and T. Schnelle (eds) *Cognition and Fact – Materials on Ludwig Fleck*, Dordrecht: D. Reidel Publishing.

Flynn, R. (1992) 'Managed Markets: Consumers and Producers in the National Health Service' in R. Burrows and C. Marsh (eds) *Consumption and Class: Divisions and Change*, London: Macmillan.

Foucault, M. (1976) *The Birth of the Clinic: An Archaeology of Medical Perception*, London, Tavistock.

Foucault, M. (1977) *Discipline and Punish*, Harmondsworth, Penguin.

Frankel, S., Davison, C. and Davey Smith, G. (1991) 'Lay Epidemiology and the Rationality of Responses to Health Education', *British Journal of General Practice*, 41, 428–38.

Frankenberg, R. (1992) 'The Other Who is Also the Same: The Relevance of Epidemics in Space and Time for Prevention of HIV Infection', *International Journal of Health Services*, 22, 1, 73–88.

Gabb, S. (1990) *Smoking and its Enemies*, London: FOREST Publications.

Gabe, J., Calnan, M. and Bury, M. (eds) (1991) *The Sociology of the Health Service*, London: Routledge.

Garfinkel, L. (1981) 'Time Trends in Lung Cancer Mortality Among Non-Smokers and a Note on Passive Smoking', *Journal of the National Cancer Institute*, 66, 6, 1061–6.

Gattas, J. T. *et al.* (1986) 'Leisure and Lifestyles: Towards a Research Agenda', *Society and Leisure*, 9, 2, 529–39.

General Dental Council (1989) *Professional Conduct and Fitness to Practise*, November, paras 23 and 24.

General Medical Services Committee (1993) *The New Health Promotion Package*, London: GMSC British Medical Association.

Gerhardt, U. (1987) 'Parsons, Role Theory, and Health Interaction' in G. Scrambler (ed.) *Sociological Theory and Medical Sociology*, London: Tavistock.

Gibson, H. B. (1992) *The Emotional and Sexual Lives of Older People*, London: Chapman and Hall.

Giddens, A. (1982) 'Hermeneutics and Social Theory' in A. Giddens, *Profiles and Critiques in Social Theory*, London: Macmillan.

Giddens, A. (1990) *The Consequences of Modernity*, Cambridge: Polity Press.

Giddens, A. (1991) *Modernity and Self-Identity: Self and Society in the Late Modern Age*, Cambridge: Polity.

Giddens, A. (1992) *The Transformation of Intimacy*, Cambridge: Polity.

Gifford, S. M. (1986) 'The Meaning of Lumps – A Case Study in the Ambiguities of Risk' in C. Janes, R. Stall and S. M. Gifford (eds), *Anthropology and Epidemiology*, Dordrecht: D. Reidel Publishing.

Gilbert, N. and Mulkay, M. (1984) *Opening Pandora's Box*, Cambridge: Cambridge University Press.

Gillis, A. J. (1993) 'Determinants of a Health Promoting Lifestyle: An Integrative Review', *Journal of Advanced Nursing*, 18, 3, 345–53.

Glassner, B. (1989) 'Fitness and the Postmodern Self', *Journal of Health and Social Behaviour*, 30, 180–91.

Glassner, B. (1992) *Bodies: The Tyranny of Perfection*, Los Angeles: Lowell House.

Godfrey, C., Hardman, G. and Maynard, A. (1989) *Priorities for Health Promotion: An Economic Approach*, Discussion Paper 59, York: Centre of Health Economics.

Goffman, E. (1968a) *Asylums: Essays on The Social Situation of Mental Patients and Other Inmates*, Harmondsworth: Penguin.

Goffman, E. (1968b) *Stigma: Notes on The Management of Spoiled Identity*, Harmondsworth: Penguin.

Goldwyn, R. (1985) 'Plastic Surgeons on the Make', *Plastic and Reconstructive Surgery*, 75, 251–2.

Gostin, L. (1986) 'The Future of Communicable Disease Control: Toward a New Concept in Public Health Law', *The Milbank Quarterly*, 64 (Supplement), 1.

Grace, V. M. (1991) 'The Marketing of Empowerment and the Construction of the Health Consumer: A Critique of Health Promotion', *International Journal of Health Services*, 21, 2, 329–43.

Graham, H. (1979) 'Prevention and Health: Every Mother's Business, A Comment on Child Health Policies in the 1970s' in C. Harris (ed.) *Sociology of the Family: New Directions for British Sociology*, University of Keele. Sociological Review Monograph 28.

Graham, H. (1984) *Women, Health and the Family*, Brighton: Harvester Wheatsheaf.

Graham, H. (1987) 'Women's Smoking and Family Health', *Social Science and Medicine*, 25, 1, 47–56.

Graham, H. (1988) 'Women and Smoking in the UK: The Implications for Health Promotion', *Health Promotion*, 4, 371–82.

Graham, H. J. and Firth, J. (1992) 'Home Accidents in Older People: The Role of the Primary Health Care Team', *British Medical Journal*, 305, 30–2.

Green, J. (1992a) 'The Medico-Legal Production of Fatal Accidents', *Sociology of Health and Illness*, 14, 373–90.

Green, J. (1992b) 'Some Problems in the Development of a Sociology of Accidents' in S. Scott, G. Williams, S. Platt and H. Thomas (eds) *Private Risks and Public Dangers*, Aldershot: Avebury.

Green, J. (1994) *Risk, Rationality and Misfortune: Towards a Sociology of Accidents*, Unpublished PhD Thesis, University of London.

Greenberg, R. A., Bauman, K. E., Strecher, V. J. et al. (1991) 'Passive Smoking During the First Year of Life', *American Journal of Public Health*, 81, 7, 850–3.

Group Against Smoking in Public (GASP) (1982) *Passive Smoking: The Facts*, Bristol: Avon Area Health Authority Education Service.

Gubrium, J. F. (1986) *Oldtimers and Alzheimer's: The Descriptive Organisation of Senility*, Greenwich, Conn. and London: JAI Press.

Gubrium, J. F. and Brandon Wallace, J. (1990) 'Who Theorises Age?', *Ageing and Society*, 10, 131–49.

Gustafsson, U. and Nettleton, S. (1992) 'The Health of Two Nations: National Strategies for Public Health and Health Promotion in England and Sweden', *International Journal of Sociology and Social Policy*, 12, 3, 1–25.

Hacking, I. (1975) *The Emergence of Probability*, Cambridge: Cambridge University Press.

Hacking, I. (1990) *The Taming of Chance*, Cambridge: Cambridge University Press.

Hahn, R. A. and Kleinman, A. (1983) 'Biomedical Practice and Anthropological Theory', *Annual Review of Anthropology*, 12, 305–33.

Hald, A. (1990) *A History of Probability and Statistics and Their Applications Before 1750*, New York: Wiley and Sons.

Hall, S., Held, D. and McGrew, T. (eds) (1992) *Modernity and Its Futures*, Cambridge: Polity.

Ham, C. (1984) 'Saving Lives or Saving Money – The Two Crises in the NHS' in P. Draper and T. Smart (eds) *Health and the Economy – The NHS Crisis in Perspective*, Unit for the Study of Health Policy, Guy's Hospital Medical School.

Hancock, T. (1986) 'Lalonde and Beyond: Looking Back at *A New Perspective on the Health of Canadians*', *Health Promotion International*, 1, 1, 93–100.

Hancock, T. (1990) 'Towards Healthy and Sustainable Communities: Health,

Environment and Economy at the Local Level', Paper Presented at the Third Colloquium on Envionmental Health, Quebec, November.

Hancock, T. (1993) 'The Healthy City: From Concept to Application' in J. Davies and M. Kelly (eds) (1993) *Healthy Cities: Research and Practice*, London: Routledge.

Hastings, G. B., Ryan, H., Teer, P. and Mackintosh, A. M. (1994) 'Cigarette Advertising and Children's Smoking: Why Reg was Withdrawn', *British Medical Journal*, 309, 933–7.

Hayes, D. and Ross, C. (1986) 'Body and Mind: The Effect of Exercise, Overweight and Physical Health on Psychological Well-Being', *Journal of Health and Social Behaviour*, 27, 387–400.

Health Education Authority (HEA) (1987) *Breathing Other People's Smoke*, London: HEA.

Health Education Authority (HEA) (1991a) *Passive Smoking – Questions and Answers*, London: HEA.

Health Education Authority (HEA) (1991b) *So You Want To Stop Smoking*, London: HEA.

Health Education Board of Scotland (1992) *Strategic Plan 1992 to 1997*, Edinburgh: Health Education Board of Scotland.

Health Education Bureau (1986) *Promoting Health Through Public Policy*, Dublin: Health Education Bureau.

Health Education Council (1983) *Healthy Living: Towards a National Strategy for Health Education and Health Promotion*, London: Health Education Council.

Health Promotion Authority for Wales (1990) *Health for All in Wales*, Cardiff: Health Promotion Authority for Wales.

Health Promotion International (1986) 'Editorial – Health Promotion: Practical Ideas in Programme Implementation', *Health Promotion International*, 1, 2, 187–90.

Henley, A. (1979) *Asian Patients in Hospital and at Home*, London: Pitman Medical.

Henley, A. (1980) *Asians in Britain: Asian Names and Records*, London: DHSS/King's Fund.

Henley, A. and Clayton, J. (1982) 'What's in a Name?', *Health and Social Service Journal*, 2: 855–7.

Henwood, M. (1992) *Accident Prevention and Public Health: A study of the Annual Reports of Directors of Public Health Birmingham*, London: Royal Society for Prevention of Accidents.

Hillman, M. (1991) 'Healthy Transport Policy' in P. Draper (ed.) *Health Through Public Policy: The Greening of Public Health*, London: Greenprint.

Hirayama, T. (1981) 'Non-Smoking Wives of Heavy Smokers Have a Higher Risk of Lung Cancer: A Study from Japan', *British Medical Journal*, 282, 183–5.

Holland, J., Ramazangolu, C., Scott, S., Sharpe, S. and Thomson R.(1990) *'Don't Die of Ignorance' – I Nearly Died of Embarrassment: Condoms in Context*, London: Tuffnell Press.

Holland, J., Ramazanoglu, C., Scott, S., Sharpe, S. and Thomson, R. (1992) 'Pressure, Resistance, Empowerment: Young Women and the Negotiation of Safe Sex' in P. Aggleton, P. Davis and G. Hart (eds) *AIDS: Rights, Risk and Reason*, London: Falmer Press.

Hollyman, J. *et al.* (1986) 'Surgery for the Psyche', *British Journal of Plastic Surgery*, 39, 222–4.

Holm, L. (1993) 'Cultural and Social Acceptability of a Healthy Diet', *European Journal of Clinical Nutrition*, 47, 8, 592–9.

Horsfield, K. (1984) 'Breathing Other People's Smoke' in G. Cumming and G. Bonsignore (eds) *Smoking and the Lung*, New York and London: Plenum Press.

Humphris, G., Morrison, T. and Horne, L. (1993) 'Perceptions of Risk of HIV Infection from Regular Attenders to an Industrial Dental Service', *British Dental Journal*, 174, 371.

Hunt, S. (1989) 'The Public Health Implications of Private Cars' in C. J. Martin and D. V. McQueen (eds) *Readings for a New Public Health*, Edinburgh: Edinburgh University Press.

Hunt, S. M., J. McEwen and S. P. McKenna (1985) *Measuring Heath Status*, London: Croom Helm.

Illich, I. (1976) *Medical Nemesis: The Expropriation of Health*, New York: Pantheon.

Independent Scientific Committee on Smoking and Health (ISCSH) (1988) *Fourth Report of the Independent Scientific Committee on Smoking and Health*, London: HMSO.

Jackson, P. (1994) 'Passive Smoking and Ill-Health: Practice and Process in the Production of Medical Knowledge', *Sociology of Health and Illness*, 16, 4.

Jacobson, B. (1986) *Beating the Ladykillers: Women and Smoking*, London: Pluto Press.

Jerrome, D. (1992) *Good Company: An Anthropological Study of People in Groups*, Edinburgh: Edinburgh University Press.

Johnson, M. (1984) 'Ethnic Minorities and Health', *Journal of the Royal College of Physicians of London*, 18, 4, 228–30.

Joliff, A. S., Gilchrist, V. J. and Bourget, C. C. (1992) 'The Impact of a Patient Survey or a Physician Reminder on the Provision of Adolescent Preventive Health Care', *Journal of Family Practice*, 35, 6, 655–9.

Jones, E. (1986) 'Cosmetic Surgery', *Essence*, April, 36–41.

Kalick, S. M. (1978) 'Towards an Interdisciplinary Psychology of Appearances', *Psychiatry*, 41, 243–53.

Kaplan, G. (1986) 'Putting on a Happier Face', *Nation's Business*, 74, 40–1.

Kelleher, C. (1993) *Measures to Promote Health and Autonomy For Older People: A Position Paper*, Publication No. 26, Dublin: The National Council for The Elderly.

Kellner, D. (1992) 'Popular Culture and the Construction of Postmodern Identity' in S. Lash and J. Friedman (eds) *Modernity and Identity*, Oxford: Blackwell.

Kelly, M P. (1989) 'Some Problems in Health Promotion Research', *Health Promotion*, 4, 317–30.

Kelly, M. P. (1990) 'Behavioural Change and the Stress Coping Paradigm: Some Comments on Modelling the European Code on Avoiding Cancer', *Journal of Public Health Medicine*, 12, 105–8.

Kelly, M. P. (1992) 'Health Promotion in Primary Care: Taking Account of the Patient's Point of View', *Journal of Advanced Nursing*, 17, 11, 1291–6.

Kelly, M. P. and Charlton, B. G. (1992) 'Health Promotion: Time for a New Philosophy?', *British Journal of General Practice*, June, 223–4.

Kelly, M. P., Charlton, B. G. and Hanlon, P. (1993a) 'The Four Levels of Health Promotion: An Integrated Approach', *Public Health*, 107, 319–26.

Kelly, M. P., Davies, J. K. and Charlton, B. G. (1993b) 'Healthy Cities: A Modern Problem or a Post-modern Solution' in J. Davies and M. Kelly (eds) (1993) *Healthy Cities: Research and Practice*, London: Routledge.

Kenner, C. (1985) *No Time for Women*, London: Pandora Press.

Khakhulina, L. A. (1984) 'Indicators for the Interrelated Study of Living Standard and Lifestyle', *Social Indicators Research* (Netherlands), 14, 3, 287–93.

Kickbusch, I. (1986) 'Health Promotion: A Global Perspective', *Canadian Journal of Public Health*, 77, 5, 321–6.

King's Fund (1988) *The Nation's Health – A Strategy for the 1990's*, London: King's Fund.

Klein, R. (1993) *Cigarettes are Sublime*, Durham, N. C.: Duke University Press.

Kleinfield, N. (1986) 'The Ever-Fatter Business of Thinness', *The New York Times*, 7 September.

Kokeny, M. (1987) *Promoting Health in Hungary*, Council of Ministers of the Hungarian People's Republic, Budapest: Central Statistical Office.

Krauss Whitbourne, S. K. (1985) *The Ageing Body: Physiological Changes and Psychological Consequences*, New York: Springer-Verlag.

Kuh, D. and Davey Smith G. (1993) 'When is Mortality Risk Determined? – Historical Insights into a Current Debate', *Social History of Medicine*, 6, 101–23.

Kuhn, T. S. (1970) *The Structure of Scientific Revolutions* (2nd edn), Chicago: University of Chicago Press.

Lake District Search and Mountain Rescue Association (LDSAMRA) (1992) *Mountain Accidents 1991*, Kendal: Lake District Mountain Rescue Association.

Lalonde, M. (1974) *A New Perspective on the Health of Canadians*, Ottawa: Information Canada.

Land, H. and Rose, H. (1985) 'Compulsory Altruism for Some or an Altruistic Society for All?' in P. Bean, J. Ferris and D.K. Whymes (eds) *In Defense of Welfare*, London: Tavistock.

Lash, S. and Urry, J. (1994) *Economies of Signs and Space*, London: Sage.

Lastovicka, J. L. and Joachminsthaler, E. A. (1988) 'Improving the Detection of Personality-Behaviour Relationships in Consumer Research', *Journal of Consumer Research*, 14, 4, 583–7.

Latour, B. and Woolgar, S. (1979) *Laboratory Life*, Beverly Hills: Sage.

Le Fanu, J. (1986) 'Diet and Disease – Nonsense and Nonscience' in D. Anderson (ed.) *A Diet of Reason*, London: Social Affairs Unit.

Lee, P. N. (1984) 'Passive Smoking' in G. Cumming and G. Bonsignore (eds) *Smoking and the Lung*, London: Plenum Press.

Lee, P. N. (1988) *Misclassification of Smoking Habits and Passive Smoking*, Berlin: Springer-Verlag.

Lee, P. N. (1992) *Environmental Tobacco Smoke and Mortality*, Basel and Munich: Karger.

Lee, P. N., Chamberlain, J. and Alderson, M. R. (1986) 'Relationship of Passive Smoking to Risk of Lung Cancer and Other Smoking-Associated Diseases', *British Journal of Cancer*, 54, 97–105.

Lees. S. (1986) *Losing Out: Sexuality and Adolescent Girls*, London: Hutchinson.

Leeson, J. and Gray, J. (1978) *Women and Medicine*, London: Tavistock.

Lefebvre, C. (1992) 'Social Marketing Health Promotion' in R. Bunton and G. Macdonald (eds) *Health Promotion: Disciplines and Diversity*, London: Routledge.

Lefebvre, C., Craig, R. and Flora, J. A. (1988) 'Social Marketing and Public Health Intervention', *Health Education Quarterly*, 15, 3.

Lefton, D. (1985) 'Ads Entice Patients to Cosmetic Surgery', *American Medical News*, 28, 6 September, 3, 17.

Leith W. (1992) 'Reg on Advertising: "You Can't Get Any Worse Than Me" ', *Independent on Sunday*, 29 November.

Lemert, C. (1992) 'General Social Theory: Irony, Post, Modernism' in S. Seidman and D. G. Wagner (eds) *Post-Modernism and Social Theory*, Oxford: Blackwell.

Lemert, E. M. (1951) *Social Pathology: A Systematic Approach to The Study of Sociopathic Behaviour*, New York: Mcgraw-Hill.

Lemert, E. M. (1967) 'The Concept of Secondary Deviation' in E. M. Lemert, *Human Deviance, Social Problems and Social Control*, Englewood Cliffs, N.J.: Prentice-Hall.

Lewis, J. (1986) *What Price Community Medicine? The Philosophy and Practice of Public Health 1918–1980*, Brighton: Wheatsheaf.

Lippert, A. (1978) 'Weight Watchers: Think Thin and Grow Fat', *Nation's Business*, September.

Lister, R. (1990) 'Women, Economic Dependency and Citizenship', *Journal of Social Policy*, 19, 4, 445–67.

Loney, M. (1983) *Community Against Government. The British Community Development Project 1968–1978: A Study in Government Incompetence*, London: Heinemann.

Lowy, I. (1988) 'Ludwig Fleck on the Social Construction of Medical Knowledge', *Sociology of Health and Illness*, 10, 2, 133–55.

Lupton, D. (1994) *Medicine as Culture: Illness, Disease and the Body in Western Societies*, London: Sage.

Lyotard, J. F. (1984) *The Post-Modern Condition: A Report on Knowledge*, Translated by G. Bennington and B. Mascum, Manchester: Manchester University Press.

Macintyre, S. (1976) 'Old Age as a Social Problem: Some Historical Notes on the British Experience', Paper Presented to the Annual Conference of The British Sociological Association, 1976. A version appears as 'Old Age as a Social Problem' in R. Dingwall, C. Heath, M. Reid and M. Stacy (eds) *Health Care and Health Knowledge*, London: Croom Helm.

McKnight, J. L. (1985) 'Health and Empowerment', *Canadian Journal of Public Health*, 76 (Supplement), 37–8.

McLennan, A. H. (1993) 'Running a Menopausal Clinic', *Baillieres Clinical and Endocrinological Metabolism*, 7, 1, 243–53.

McQueen, D. (1989) 'Thoughts on the Ideological Origins of Health Promotion', *Health Promotion*, 4, 4, 339–42.

Mahler, H. (1984) 'Address to the Ottawa Conference', *Health Promotion International*, 4, 1–2.

Mahler, M. (1986) 'Editorial Introduction: Towards a New Public Health', *Health Promotion*, 1, 1.

Manos, R. K. (1985) *Social Marketing: A New Imperative for Public Health*, New York: Praeger.

Mares, P., Henley, A. and Baxter, C. (1985) *Health Care in Multiracial Britain*, Cambridge: Health Education Council.

Marsh, S. and McKay, S. (1994) *Poor Smokers*, London: Policy Studies Institute.

Martin, C. J. and McQueen, D. V. (1989) *Readings for a New Public Health*, Edinburgh: Edinburgh University Press.

Marx, K. (1962) *Capital: A Critique of Political Economy*, Moscow: Foreign Languages Publishing House.

Marx, K. and Engels, F. (1970) *The German Ideology* (Edited by C. J. Arthur), London: Lawrence and Wishart.

Matza, D. (1969) *Becoming Deviant*, Englewood Cliffs, NJ: Prentice-Hall.

Maycock, G., Lockwood, C. R. and Lester, J. F. (1991) *The Accident Liability of Car Drivers*, Research Report 315, London: HMSO.

Melia, R. J. M., Morrell, D. C., Swann, A. and Bartholomew, J. (1989) 'A Health Visitor Investigation of Home Accidents in Pre-School Children', *Health Visitor*, 62, 181–3.

Melvin, B. (1987) 'Promoting Health by Example', *Nursing Times*, 83, 17.

Mennell, S., Murcott, A. and van Otterloo, A. H. (1992) *The Sociology of Food*, London: Sage.

Merton, R. (1973) *The Sociology of Science*, Chicago: University of Chicago Press.

Miles, A. (1991) *Women, Health and Medicine*, Milton Keynes, Open University Press.

Miller, L. (1979) 'Towards a Classification of Ageing Behaviours', *The Gerontologist*, 19, 3, 283–90.

Miller, L. (1987) 'The Professional Construction of Ageing', *Journal of Gerontological Social Work*, 10, 3/4, 141–53.

Milton Keynes Health Authority (1987) *District Profile*, Milton Keynes Health Authority.

Mills, M. (ed.) (1993) *Prevention, Health and British Politics*, Aldershot: Avebury.

Mindell, J. (1992) 'Review: Direct Tobacco Advertising and its Impact on Children', *Journal of Smoking-Related Diseases*, 3, 3, 275–84.

Morley, D., Rolide, J. and Williams, G. (1987) *Practising Health for All*, Oxford: Oxford University Press.

Morris, J. (1993) *Independent Lives: Community Care and Disabled People*, London: Macmillan.

Mulkay, M. (1979) *Science and the Sociology of Knowledge*, London: George Allen and Unwin.

Mulkay, M. (1984) 'Knowledge and Utility: Implications for the Sociology of Knowledge' in N. Stehr and V. Meja (eds) *Society and Knowledge: Contemporary Perspectives in the Sociology of Knowledge*, New Brunswick: Transaction Books.

Mullen K. (1992) 'A Question of Balance: Health Behaviour and Work Context Among Male Glaswegians', *Sociology of Health and Illness*, 14, 1, 73–97.

Murray, R. (1989) 'Fordism and Post-Fordism' in S. Hall and M. Jacques (eds) *New Times*, London: Lawrence and Wishart.

Naidoo, J. (1986) 'Limits to Individualism' in S. Rodmell and A. Watt (eds) *The Politics of Health Education*, London: Routledge and Kegan Paul.

National Association of Health Authorities and the Royal Society for the Prevention of Accidents (1990) *Action on Accidents*, Birmingham: National Association of Health Authorities.

National Health Service Management Executive (1992) *Women in the NHS: An Implementation Guide to Opportunity 2000*, London: Department of Health.

National Health Service Management Executive (1993) *Better Living–Better Lives*, Leeds: NHS Management Executive.

Nelkin, D. and Tancredi, L. (1989) *Dangerous Diagnostics – The Social Power of Biological Information*, New York: Basic Books.

Nettleton, S. (1986) 'Understanding Dental Health Beliefs: An Introduction to Ethnography', *British Dental Journal*, 161, 4, 145–7.

Nettleton, S. (1991) 'Wisdom, Diligence and Teeth: Discursive Practices and the Creation of Mothers', *Sociology of Health and Illness*, 13, 1, 98–111.

Nettleton, S. (1992) *Power, Pain and Dentistry*, Buckingham: Open University Press.

Nettleton, S. (1995) *The Sociology of Health and Illness*, Cambridge: Polity.

Nettleton, S. and Burrows, R. (1994) 'From Bodies in Hospitals to People in the

Community: A Theoretical Analysis of the Relocation of Health Care', *Care in Place*, 1, 2, 3–13.

Nietzsche, F. (1974) *The Gay Science*, New York: Random House.

Noack, H. (1987) 'Concepts of Health and Health Promotion' in T. Abelin, Z. J. Brzezinski and V.D.L. Carstairs (eds) *Measurement in Health Promotion and Protection*, Copenhagen: World Health Organisation.

Northrup, B. (1987) 'Doctors Doing Cosmetic Work Scrap Over Turf', *The Wall Street Journal*, 26 February, 25.

No Smoking Day (1994) *Breathtaking*, Leaflet Promoting National No Smoking Day, London.

Novak, J. C. (1988) 'The Social Mandate and Historical Basis for Nursing's Role in Health Promotion', *Journal of Professional Nursing*, 4, 2, 80–7.

Oakley, A. (1984) *The Captured Womb: A History of the Medical Care of Pregnant Women*, Oxford: Blackwell.

Oakley, A. (1989) 'Smoking in Pregnancy: Smoke Screen or Risk Factor? Towards a Materialistic Analysis', *Sociology of Health and Illness*, 11, 311–55.

O'Brien, M. (1992) 'Is This Your Lifestyle? Sociology and the Synthetic Consumer', *Occasional Papers in Sociology and Social Research*, No. 3, Department of Sociology, University of Surrey.

Open University (1992–3) *Health and Wellbeing*, A Second Level Course Presented in Three Workbooks: 1 *Health as a Contested Concept*; 2 *Debates and Decisions in Everyday Health*; and 3 *Health on a Wider Agenda*, Milton Keynes: The Open University.

Ornish, D., Brown, S. E., Scherwitz, L. W., Billings, J. H. and Armstrong, W. T. (1990) 'Can Lifestyle Changes Reverse Coronary Heart Disease? The Lifestyle Heart Trial', *Lancet*, 336, 129–33.

Orr, J. (1988) 'Women's Health: A Nursing Perspective' in R. White (ed.) *Political Issues in Nursing: Past, Present and Future*, Chichester: John Wiley and Sons.

Oxford Regional Health Authority (1987) *Health for All in the Oxford Region: A Health Promotion Review*, Oxford Regional Health Authority.

Oxford Universal Dictionary Illustrated (1965) revised edn, Oxford: Clarendon Press.

Parish, R. (1986) *The Practical Asects of Programme Implementation*, Report of a WHO Seminar, Copenhagen: World Health Organisation.

Parsons, T. (1951) *The Social System*, Glencoe: Free Press.

Parsons, T. (1958) 'Definitions of Health and Illness in the Light of American Values and Social Structure' in E. Jaco (ed.) *Patients, Physicians, and Illness*, New York: Free Press.

Parsons, T. (1975) 'The Sick Role and the Role of the Physician Reconsidered', *Health and Society*, 53, 3.

Patton, C. (1990) *Inventing AIDS*, London: Routledge.

Pearson, K. (1897) *The Chances of Death and Other Studies in Evolution* (2 Vols), London: Edward Arnold.

Pearson, M. (1986) 'Racist Notions of Ethnicity and Culture in Health Education' in S. Rodmell and A. Watt (eds) *The Politics of Health Education*, London: Routledge and Kegan Paul.

Pearson, M. (1989) 'Sociology of Race and Health' in K. Cruikshank and D. Beeves (eds) *Ethnic Factors in Health and Disease*, London: Wright.

Pembrokeshire Health Authority (1988) *Manual for the Primary Health Care Facilitator Project*, Pembrokeshire Health Authority.

Phillimore, P., Beattie, A. and Townsend, P. (1994) 'Widening Inequality of Health in Northern England, 1981 – 91' *British Medical Journal*, 308, 1125–8.

Picavet, Fr. (1971) *Les idéologues*, New York: Burt Franklin.

Pill, R. and Stott, N. C. H. (1982) 'Concepts of Illness Causation and Responsibility: Some Preliminary Data from a Sample of Working Class Mothers', *Social Science and Medicine*, 16, 43–52.

Pill, R., Peters, T. J. and Robling, M. R. (1993) 'Factors Associated with Health Behaviour Among Mothers of Lower Socio-Economic Status', *Social Science and Medicine*, 36, 9, 1137–44.

Plant, M. and Plant, M. (1992) *The Risk Takers*, London: Routledge.

Plummer, K. (1988) 'Organising AIDS' in P. Aggleton and H. Homans (eds) *Social Aspects of AIDS*, London: Falmer Press.

Polnay, L. (1992) 'Is Neglect Neglected?' in J. Sibert (ed.) *Accidents and Emergencies in Childhood*, London: Royal College of Physicians.

Popay, J. and Young, A. (eds) (1993) *Reducing Accidental Death and Injury in Children*, A Report Produced for the North West Regional Health Authority Public Health Working Group on Child Accidents, Manchester: Public Health Resources Centre.

Popper, K. (1959) *The Logic of Scientific Discovery*, London: Hutchinson.

Porritt, J. (1990) *Seeing Green: The Politics of Ecology Explained*, Blackwell: Oxford.

Prashar, U., Anoniu, E. and Brozovic, H. (1985) *Sickle Cell Anaemia – Who Cares?* London: Runnymede Trust.

Puska, P. *et al.* (1985) 'The Community Based Strategy to Prevent Coronary Heart Disease: Conclusions from the Ten Years of the North Karelia Project', *Annual Reviews of Public Health*, 36, 2.

Radical Statistics Health Group (RSHG) (1987) 'Health Education – Blaming the Victim?' in *Facing the Figures – What is Really Happening in the NHS?*, London: Radical Statistics.

Rappaport, J. (1977) 'Terms of Empowerment/Exemplars of Prevention: Toward a Theory for Community Psychology', *American Journal of Community Psychology*, 15, 121–45.

Rawson, D. and Grigg, C. (1988) *Purpose and Practice in Health Education*, London: South Bank Polytechnic/Health Education Authority.

Reich, J. (1969) 'The Surgery of Appearance', *Medical Journal of Australia*, 2, 5–13.

Repace. J. L. and Lowrey, A. H. (1980) 'Indoor Air Pollution, Tobacco Smoke and Public Health', *Science*, 208, 464–72.

Research Unit in Health and Behaviour Change (1989) *Changing the Public Health*, Chichester: John Wiley and Sons.

Rheingold, H. (1994) *The Virtual Community: Finding Connection in a Computerized World*, London: Secker and Warburg.

Rice, B. (1988) 'The Selling of Lifestyles', *Psychology Today*, 22, 3, 46–50.

Rich, A. (1977) *Of Woman Born*, London: Virago.

Ritenbaugh, C. (1982) 'Obesity as a Culture-Bound Syndrome', *Culture, Medicine and Psychiatry*, 6, 347–61.

Roberts, H. (ed) (1990) *Women's Health Counts*, London: Routledge.

Roberts, H., Smith, S. and Bryce, C. (1993) 'Prevention is Better . . .' *Sociology of Health and Illness*, 15, 447–63.

Roberts, H., Smith, S. and Lloyd, M. (1992) 'Safety as Social Value: A Community Approach' in S. Scott, G. Williams, S. Platt and H. Thomas (eds) *Private Risks and Public Dangers*, Aldershot: Avebury.

Roberts, S. E. (1992) *Healthy Participation: An Evaluative Study of the Hartcliffe*

Health and Environment Action Group, A Community Development Project in Bristol, Unpublished MSc Dissertation, University of West England, Bristol.

Rocheron, Y. (1988) 'The Asian Mother and Baby Campaign: the Construction of Ethnic Minorities' Health Needs', *Critical Social Policy*, 22: 4–23.

Rodmell, S. and Watt, A. (eds) (1986) *The Politics of Health Education*, London: Routledge and Kegan Paul.

Rorty, R. (1982) 'Method, Social Science and Social Hope' in R. Rorty (1982) *Consequences of Pragmatism: Essays 1972–80*, Brighton: Harvester Press.

Rose, N. (1990) *Governing the Soul: The Shaping of the Private Self*, London: Routledge.

Rosenthal, S. (1982) 'Malpractice: Through the Looking Glass', *Annals of Plastic and Reconstructive Surgery*, 9, 326–9.

Roszak, T. (1981) *Person/Planet*, St Albans: Granada.

Rotter, J. (1982) *The Development and Application of Social Learning Theory*, New York: Praeger.

Royal College of Physicians (1962) *Smoking and Health*, London: Report of the Royal College of Physicians.

Royal Ulster Constabulary (1992) *Road Traffic Accident Statistics 1991*, Belfast: HMSO.

Rucker, R., Sirius, R. U. and Queen Mu (1993) *Mondo 2000: A User's Guide to the New Edge*, London: Thames and Hudson.

Salter, B. (1993) 'Public Image Limited', *Health Service Journal*, 15 July.

Saunders, P. (1984) 'Beyond Housing Classes', *International Journal of Urban and Regional Research*, 2, 233–51.

Savage, M. and Warde, A. (1993) *Urban Sociology, Capitalism and Modernity*, Basingstoke: Macmillan.

Savage, M., Barlow, J., Dickens, P. and Fielding, T. (1992) *Property, Bureaucracy and Culture: Middle Class Formation in Contemporary Britain*, London: Routledge.

Scheiner, A. (1986) 'My Face-Lift: A Cautionary Tale', *Ms*, 58, 63, 81–2 November.

Scheper-Hughes, N. and Lock, M. (1987) 'The Mindful Body – A Prolegomenon to Future Work in Medical Anthropology', *Medical Anthropology Quarterly*, 1, 6–41.

Schnabel, P. (1992) 'Down and Out: Social Marginality and Homelessness', *International Journal of Social Psychiatry*, 38, 1, 59–67.

Schumacher, F. (1974) *Small is Beautiful*, Tunbridge Wells: Abacus.

Schwarz, J. (1988) 'Bitestyles of the Rich and Famous', *American Demographics*, 9.

Schwartz, M., Savage, W., George, J. and Emohare, L. (1989) 'Women's Knowledge and Experience of Cervical Screening: A Failure of Health Education and Medical Organisation', *Community Medicine*, 45, 279–89.

Scott, S. and Morgan, D. (eds) (1993) *Body Matters: Essays on the Sociology of the Body*, London: Falmer Press.

Scott, S., Williams, G., Platt, S. and Thomas, H. (eds) (1992) *Private Risks and Public Dangers*, Aldershot: Avebury.

Scott-Samuel, A. (1989) 'Building the New Public Health: A Public Health Alliance and a New Social Epidemiology' in C.J. Martin and D.V. McQueen, *Readings for a New Public Health*, Edinburgh: Edinburgh University Press.

Seidman, S. and Wagner, D. G. (eds) (1992) *Post-Modernism and Social Theory*, Oxford: Blackwell.

Shama, A. (1988) 'The Voluntary Simplicity Consumer: A Comparative Study', *Psychological Reports*, 63, 3, 859–69.

Sheiham, H. and Quick, A. (1982) *The Rickets Report*, London: Harringay Community Health Council and Community Relations Council.

Sheldon, T. (1993) 'Vive la Difference?', *Health Service Journal*, 15 July.

Shephard, R. J. (1982) *The Risks of Passive Smoking*, London: Croom Helm.

Shilling, C. (1993) *The Body and Social Theory*, London: Sage.

Skrabanek, P. (1988) 'Controversy Over Mammography Screening: The Case Against', *British Medical Journal*, 300, 916–18.

Skrabanek, P. (1991) 'Risk Factor Epidemiology: Science or Non-Science' in Social Affairs Unit, *Health, Lifestyle and Environment: Countering the Panic*, London: Social Affairs Unit.

Skrabanek, P. (1992) 'Politics and Ideology of Health Promotion', *Medical Audit News*, 1992, 2, 82–3.

Smart, C. (1992) *Regulating Womanhood: Historical Essays on Marriage, Motherhood and Sexuality*, London: Routledge.

Smithson, M (1985) 'Toward a Social Theory of Ignorance', *Journal for the Theory of Social Behaviour*, 15, 2.

Snyder, J. R. (1988) 'Translator's Introduction' in G. Vattimo (1988) *The End of Modernity: Nihilism and Hermeneutics in Post-Modern Culture*, Cambridge: Polity.

Sobel, M. E. (1981) *Lifestyle and Social Structure: Concepts, Definitions, Analyses*, New York: Academic Press.

Social Affairs Unit (1991) *Health, Lifestyle and Environment: Countering the Panic*, London: Social Affairs Unit.

Speer, F. (1968) 'Tobacco and the Non-Smoker', *Archives of Environmental Health*, 16, 443–6.

Spiegel, C. N. and Lindaman, F. C. (1977) 'Children Can't Fly: A Program to Prevent Childhood Morbidity and Mortality from Window Falls', *American Journal of Public Health*, 67, 1143–7.

Stacey, M. (1991) 'Medical Sociology and Health Policy: An Historical Overview' in J. Gabe, M. Calnan and M. Bury (eds) *The Sociology of the Health Service*, London: Routledge.

Stehr, N. and Meja, V. (eds) (1984) *Society and Knowledge – Contemporary Perspectives in the Sociology of Knowledge*, New Brunswick: Transaction Books.

Stephens, J. (1980) *Loners, Losers and Lovers: Elderly Tenants in A Slum Hotel*, Seattle and London: University of Washington Press.

Sterling, T. (1978) 'Does Smoking Kill Workers or Does Work Kill Smokers? – The Mutual Relationship Between Smoking, Occupation and Respiratory Disease', *International Journal of Health Services*, 8, 437–52.

Stevenson, H. M. and Burke, M. (1991) 'Bureaucratic Logic in New Social Movement Clothing: The Limits of Health Promotion Research', *Health Promotion International*, 6, 281–96.

Stockport Area Health Authority (1980) *Strategy for the Development of the Health Education Service in Stockport*, Stockport Area Health Authority Health Education Service.

Stone, D. (1991) 'Preventing Accidents – A High Priority Target', *Medical Monitor*, 24 May, 61–5.

Stott, N. (1994) 'Screening for Cardiovascular Risk in General Practice' *British Medical Journal*, 308, 29, 285–6.

Stott, N. C. and Pill, R. M. (1990) ' "Advise Yes, Dictate, No". Patients' Views on Health Promotion in the Consultation', *Family Practitioner*, 7, 2, 125–31.

Strauss, R. (1957) 'The Nature and Status of Medical Sociology', *American Sociological Review*, 22, 200–4.

Sutherland, R. (1992) 'Preventing Child Traffic Injuries' in J. Sibert (ed.) *Accidents and Emergencies in Childhood*, London: Royal College of Physicians.

Taylor, P. (1985) *The Smoke Ring*, London: Sphere Books.

Tesh, S. N. (1988) *Hidden Arguments: Political Ideology and Disease Prevention Policy*, New Brunswick: Rutgers University Press.

Thompson, J. and Brown, B. (1990) *Screening and Health Promotion: Seminar Report*, Blackpool: Wyre and Fylde Health Authority.

Thorogood, N. (1990) 'Caribbean Home Remedies and their Importance for Black Women's Health Care in Britain' in P. Abbott and G. Payne (eds) *New Directions in the Sociology of Health*, London: Falmer Press.

Thorogood, N. (1992a) 'Sex Education as Social Control', *Critical Public Health*, 3, 2, 43–50.

Thorogood, N. (1992b) 'What is the Relevance of Sociology for Health Promotion?' in R. Bunton and G. MacDonald (eds) *Health Promotion: Disciplines and Diversity*, London: Routledge.

Tinker, A. (1992) *Elderly People in Modern Society*, 3rd edn, London and New York: Longman.

Tombs, S. (1991) 'Injury and Ill Health in the Chemical Industry: Decentering the Accident Prone Victim', *Industrial Crisis Quarterly*, 5, 59–75.

Tones, B. K. (1986) 'Health Education and the Ideology of Health Promotion: A Review of Alternative Approaches', *Health Education Research*, 1, 3–12.

Townsend, B. and Riche, M. F. (1987) 'Two Paychecks and Seven Lifestyles: Here are the Most Important Segments of a Most Desirable Consumer Group', *American Demographics*, 9, 24–30.

Townsend, P., Davidson, N. and Whitehead, M. (eds) (1988) *The Black Report and the Health Divide*, Harmondsworth: Penguin.

Townsend, P., Phillimore, P. and Beattie, A. (1988) *Health and Deprivation: Inequality and the North*, London: Routledge.

Trichopolous, D., Kalandidi, A., Sparros, L. and MacMahon, B. (1981) 'Lung Cancer and Passive Smoking', *International Journal of Cancer*, 27, 1–4.

Tsouros, A. and Draper, R. A. (1993) 'The Healthy Cities Project: New Developments and Research Needs' in J. Davies and M. Kelly (eds) (1993) *Healthy Cities: Research and Practice*, London: Routledge.

Tunon, C. (1986) 'When in Rome', *Health Education Journal*, 45, 2, 103–4.

Turner, B. S. (1991) 'Recent Developments in the Theory of the Body' in M. Featherstone, M. Hepworth and B. S. Turner (eds) *The Body: Social Processes and Cultural Theory*, London: Sage.

Turner, B. S. (1992) *Regulating Bodies: Essays in Medical Sociology*, London: Routledge.

Turner, J. (1986) 'Health for All Gains Ground', *Times Health Supplement*, 3, 7, 1 July.

Urry, J. (1990) *The Tourist Gaze: Leisure and Travel in Contemporary Societies*, London: Sage.

US Department of Health, Education and Welfare (1979) *Smoking and Health: A Report of the Surgeon General*, Public Health Service Publication 79–50066: Washington D.C.

Viscusi, W. K. (1992) *Smoking – Making the Risky Decision*, Oxford: Oxford University Press.

von Mises, R. (1939) *Probability, Statistics and Truth*, London: W. Hodge and Co.

Wagner, P. (1994) *A Sociology of Modernity: Liberty and Discipline*, London: Routledge.

Walby, S. (1994) 'Is Citizenship Gendered?', *Sociology*, 28, 2, 379–95.

Wald, N., Boreham, J., Bailey, A. *et al.* (1984) 'Urinary Cotinine as a Marker of Breathing Other People's Tobacco Smoke', *Lancet*, 28 January, 230–1.

Wang, C. (1992) 'Culture Meaning and Disability: Injury Prevention Campaigns and the Production of Stigma', *Social Science and Medicine*, 35, 9, 1093–102.

Warde, A. (1990) 'Introduction to the Sociology of Consumption', *Sociology*, 24, 1.

Warde, A. (1992) 'Notes on the Relationship Between Production and Consumption' in R. Burrows and C. Marsh (eds) *Consumption and Class: Divisions and Change*, London: Macmillan.

Warkins, P. (1991) 'Energy Comes Poisoned' in P. Draper (ed.) *Health Through Public Policy: The Greening of Public Health*, London: Greenprint.

Watney, S. (1988) 'AIDS "Moral Panic" Theory and Homophobia' in P. Aggleton and H. Homans (eds) *Social Aspects of AIDS*, London: Falmer Press.

Watt, A. (1986) 'Community Health Education: A Time for Caution?' in S. Rodmell and A. Watt, *The Politics of Health Education*, London: Routledge and Kegan Paul.

Watt, A. and Rodmell, S. (1993) 'Community Involvement in Health Promotion: Progress or Panacea?' in A. Beattie, M. Gott, L. Jones and M. Sidell (eds) *Health and Wellbeing: A Reader*, London: Macmillan.

Webb, T. and Schilling, R. (1988) *Health Promotion at Work? A Report on Health Promotion in the Workplace*, London: Health Education Authority.

Weber, M. (1930) *The Protestant Ethic and the Spirit of Capitalism* (trans. T. Parsons), London: Unwin.

Weber, M. (1947) *The Theory of Social and Economic Organizations* (Translated by A. Henderson and T. Parsons), New York: Free Press.

Weber, M. (1948) *From Max Weber: Essays in Sociology* (Edited by H. Gerth and C. W. Mills), London: Routledge and Kegan Paul.

Weber, M. (1961) *General Economic History*, London: Collier Macmillan.

Weber, M. (1963) *The Sociology of Religion*, Boston: Beacon.

Webster, S. (1991) 'The Arms Traders' in P. Draper (ed.) *Health Through Public Policy: The Greening of Public Health*, London: Greenprint.

Weeks, D. (1993) 'O5O', 20, Autumn.

Wells, N. (1987) *Women's Health Today*, London: Office of Health Economics.

Wenger, C. (1993) 'The Ageing World: Longevity, Culture and The Individual', *Generations Review*, 3, 3.

Wernick, A. (1991) *Promotional Culture: Advertising, Ideology and Symbolic Expression*, London: Sage.

White, K. (1991) 'The Sociology of Health and Illness', *Current Sociology*, 39, 2.

White, M. and Bhopal, R. (1993) 'Health Promotion for Ethnic Minorities', *HFA 2000 News*, 22, 3–5.

World Health Organisation (1946) *Constitution*, New York: WHO.

World Health Organisation (1971) *Smoking and Health*, London: DHSS.

World Health Organisation (1978) *Alma Ata 1977, Primary Health Care*, Geneva: WHO.

World Health Organisation (1981) *Regional Strategy for Attaining Health for All by the Year 2000*, Copenhagen: WHO.

World Health Organisation (1984) *Health Promotion: A Discussion Document on the Concepts and Principles*, Copenhagen: WHO.

World Health Organisation (1985) *Health for All 2000: Targets for Europe*, Copenhagen: WHO.

World Health Organisation (1986a) *Ottawa Charter for Health Promotion*, Canada: WHO. Reproduced in *Health Promotion*, 1, 1.

World Health Organisation (1986b) 'Lifestyles and Health', *Social Science and Medicine*, 22, 2, 117–24.

World Health Organisation (1988a) *Research Policies for Health For All*, Copenhagen, WHO.

World Health Organisation (1988b) *Priority Research for Health For All*, Copenhagen, WHO.

World Health Organisation (1988c) *The Adelaide Recommendations: Healthy Public Policy*, Copenhagen: WHO.

Williams, G. and Popay, J. (1994) 'Lay Knowledge and the Privilege of Experience' in J. Gabe, D. Kelleher and G. Williams (eds) *Challenging Medicine*, London: Routledge.

Williams, K. (1985) 'The High Costs of Looking Young', *Money*, April, 67–76.

Williams, R. (1990) *A Protestant Legacy: Attitudes to Death and Illness Among Older Aberdonians*, Oxford: Clarendon Press.

Williams, S., Calnan, M., Cant, S. and Coyle, J. (1993) 'All Change in the NHS: Implications of the NHS Reforms for Primary Care Prevention', *Sociology of Health and Illness*, 15, 1.

Willis, P. (1990) *Common Culture*, Milton Keynes: Open University Press.

Wilton, T. (1994) 'Feminism and the Erotics of Health Promotion' in L. Doyal, J. Naidoo and T. Wilton (eds) *Women and AIDS: Setting a Feminist Agenda*, London: Taylor and Francis.

Winchester Health Promotion Department (1989) *Annual Report*, Winchester Health Authority.

Woodward, K. (1991) *Ageing and Its Discontents: Freud and Other Fictions*, Bloomington and Indianapolis: Indiana University Press.

Yeats, W. B. (1973) [1920] 'The Second Coming' in P. Allt and R.K. Alspach (eds) *The Variorum Edition of the Poems of W.B.Yeats*, New York: Macmillan.

Young, I. (1993) 'Healthy Eating Policies in Schools: An Evaluation of Effects on Pupils' Knowledge, Attitude and Behaviour', *Health Education Journal*, 52, 3–9.

Zola, I. (1972) 'Medicine as an Institution of Social Control', *Sociological Review*, 20, 487–504.

Name index

Subject index